Nitric Oxide,
the Mighty Molecule: Its Benefits for Your Health and Well-Being

Hernan R. Chang, M.D., F.A.C.P.

ISBN: 0615532152
ISBN-13: 9780615532158
Library of Congress Control Number: 2011937690
The Mind Society, Jacksonville, FL

Printed in the United States of America

Table of Contents

1

Introduction

THE HUMAN BODY is a wonderful and fascinating conglomeration of intricate parts. It is a simple but complex synthesis of various different but related components working to keep you healthy. Some organs, such as the lungs, heart, stomach, and liver, are large and singularly important. Other body mechanisms are small and minute, seen only through the lens of a microscope.

There are muscles, tendons, and joints we can feel when we use them. Yet the body also contains microorganisms, proteins, enzymes, and other substances we cannot see or even feel. Nevertheless, they are there. If they are not present, if one small component of this system is lacking, is malfunctioning, or is present in too large a number, any manner of things can go from slightly to horribly wrong.

The various processes a body undertakes or instigates to make sure you remain healthy are numerous and complex. They may involve anywhere from a single action to hundreds of different, interrelated actions. In fact, researchers have yet to explain why and how many of these actions occur within your body. Consider DNA and the field of genetics. It is an ongoing process undertaken by scientists all over the world to locate and understand the purpose and role of each strand and component of genetic material. In unlocking the secrets of one strand, it is believed you can find information about why a disease may occur or how to suppress or cure certain illnesses or genetically based problems.

The same search for the truth is true for other materials, substances, and components that comprise the functions and make-up of the body. These include research on some that are a product of the body's need to function at its optimal level. Take, for instance, the substance of nitric oxide (NO). Scientists have long since understood how it affects the air quality. In fact, this was the focus of almost all the research on NO.

Nitric oxide is toxic when released into the air. It is produced when lightning strikes. It is also found in small amounts in the soil. Yet what NO is most famous for is nothing to laugh about. It was and is responsible for adding to the pollution known as smog—nitric oxide and nitrogen dioxide, carbon dioxide, and water, as well as a few other substances—in the ancient city of London, England, and in present-day Los Angeles. Yet it was not actually until the 1970s that researchers discovered the positive side of nitric oxide. They uncovered how this tiny molecule is capable of maintaining a healthy body. They learned that while NO in the air was a no-no, NO produced by the body was a necessity. This is the story of the mighty molecule that could and does play a vital role in keeping your body healthy. It is a tale of how a small gas can prolong your life, lower your blood pressure, alleviate the problem of erectile dysfunction, and help you with your memory.

2

Nitric Oxide:
Definition, Chemistry, and History

NITRIC OXIDE IS a relative new comer to the arsenal of medicine. For those that wish to create and maintain a healthy body it has become a new focal point. Before looking at the history of its development, it is best to understand the very basics about this essential molecule. To accomplish this it is necessary to answer the question: "What is Nitric Oxide?"

What Is Nitric Oxide?

Nitric oxide is classified as many things. It is:

1. A chemical

2. A gas

3. A biological molecule

4. A product of enzymes, particularly by the conversion of L-arginine

5. Produced in the lining (endothelium) of the blood vessels; this is scientifically referred to as endothelium nitric oxide (eNO)

While a small and simple molecule that lasts but seconds after its release, NO is a very useful gas (Fukato, Cho, and Switzer, 2000). It is also the first known gas to act as a signaling molecule within the human body (Cooke and Zimmer, 2003). This means the molecule acts as a messenger or transmitter, sending off signals to other body components or materials to perform such-and-such and act. Research since the 1980s has resulted in discovering a multitude of useful properties for NO that extend far beyond its deceivingly basic chemical composition (Bryan and Loscalzo, 2011).

Chemistry

Nitric oxide is diatomic (Butler and Nicholson, 2003). This means it consists of two atoms—in this case, nitrogen and oxygen. The symbol 'NO' indicates that the process involves the joining together of a single atom from each gas to produce it. NO also has an impaired electron.

Other characteristics include the ability to react rapidly with other molecules. NO can also diffuse using the plasma membranes to obtain its objective—to reach the target protein. It can accomplish this because it is lipophilic or attracted to fats (Garbán, 2010). This means NO is also only slightly soluble in water.

Different methods create NO within and without the body. Outside the body, NO is a colorless gas at room temperature. Inside the body, while still colorless and a gas, the source and development is the result of the coordination of different mechanisms and substances. The process is quite intricate and depends upon the source of the NO.

The method of creating NO inside the body involves an earlier action—the conversion of a specific enzyme group into NO through a process called nitric oxide synthase (NOS). This is the family of enzymes, specific to the system involved. In fact, there are at least three types of NOS families. They are those associated with:

- Endothelial cells

- Brain and nervous system cells

- Immune cells (Fried and Merrell, 1999)

The NOS family act to break down the enzymes to release the NO gas as well as citrulline into the specific system, e.g. endothelium, nervous system, immune system (Fukato, et. al., 2000). The NOS members of each system are considered either constitutive (neuronal and endothelial) or inducible. The constitutive isoforms of NOS are also called NOS1 (or nNOS) and NOS3 (or eNOS). The inducible isoform of NOS refers to the NOS (NOS2) of the immune cells and macrophages (Thomas Flores-Santana, Switzer, Wink, and Ridnour, 2010; Ganong, 2005). This is also referred to as iNOS (Garbán, 2010).

The actual production of NO involves several steps. It also engages several different substances from start to finish. While nitrites and nitrates are enzymes involved in the process, the most common and recognized producer of NO is L-arginine. NO is actually extracted from the guanidino nitrogen atoms of L-arginine (Moncada and Higgs, 1993).

ARGININE

How much is made, and when and if, is dependent upon the availability of arginine. The supply for NO production may be limited by different factors, including the presence of an NOS inhibitor such as asymmetric dimethylarginine (ADMA). Other possibilities affecting NO production from arginine are competing needs of other metabolic pathways and any alterations to the composition of arginine.

Arginine is classified as a semi-essential amino acid (Cooke, et. al., 2002). It occurs naturally within the body and in certain foods, including meats and vegetables. Arginine is actually one of the so-called "twenty-two building blocks" that comprise the basic proteins essential for every living cell to exist and thrive (Fried, et. al., 1999). It is produced in the lining of the blood vessels: the endothelium.

ENDOTHELIUM

Your body contains miles and miles of blood vessels and cavities. They run throughout and are located within the entire length of your body. Each has an outer coating as well as an inner membrane. The inner membrane is called the endothelium (Markovitch, 2006).

The endothelium is a single covering, a fibrous layer or carpet of small, plate-like cells: endothelium cells. These cells act as a lining for the blood vessel (Butler, et. al., 2003). The cells that comprise the endothelium form part of what is one of our largest organs that can be considered autocrine, paracrine, and endocrine (Von Hachling, Anker, and Bassenger, 2004). This implies a system that is able to self-stimulate to perform a specific task (autocrine), capable of arranging for actions by sending signals into a nearby area (paracrine), and able to send off any messages into the actual blood-stream (endocrine).

This action is facilitated by the extent of the system. Endothelium cells truly are spread throughout the body since they line every blood vessel (Cooke, et. al., 2003). Amazingly enough, the endothelium is not only ex-tensive, but it is also self-healing. It contains a vascular endothelial growth factor (VEGF) that helps the cells repair any damage (Sears and Sears, 2010). VEGF is a mediator and acts as a mitogen. In the former process, VEGF actually stimulates the endothelial cells, causing them to form new blood vessels. The process is called angiogenesis. Acting directly on the endothelial lining, VEGF, as a mitogen, causes the affected cells to split, dividing and multiplying. This process is called mitosis (Markovitch, 2006).

However, the processes involved in producing NO via the endothelial cells are not as simple as the make-up of the NO molecule. It is a complex proce-dure of both interrelated and independent processes (Fukato, et. al., 2000). It involves a system of integrated, independent, and balanced components of the body working together to produce it.

How It Works

The process through which NO comes into existence and performs its "mir-acles" is neither simple nor easy to explain. In fact, scientists are still looking at the entire procedure to uncover and explore such facets as dosage, trig-gers, external effects, application, and possible side-effects. To reduce it to the simplest terms possible is to ignore the intricacies of the system. Yet it is possible to strip the action down to the basics and retain the essence of the transformation.

The L-arginine nitric oxide pathway and its results can be described accordingly:

1. L-arginine is digested and utilized by the endothelial cells.

2. During the process, L-arginine breaks down into different parts.

3. To do so, L-arginine and NO require what is called a nitric oxide synthase or NOS.

4. The result is nitric oxide (NO) and another molecule, prostacyclin (Cooke, et. al., 2002).

5. NO and prostacyclin act together to maintain healthy blood vessels. NO acts upon the endothelium as a signaler—it first sends a signal to the inner smooth-muscle cells of artery walls.

6. NO also acts as a relaxer and vasodilator—it causes the artery walls to relax and enlarges or dilates the blood vessels through activation of guanylyl cyclose, which, in turn, produces cyclic guanosine monophosphate or cGMP (Esselstyn, 2008; Roizen and Oz, 2008).

7. This creates a slippery blood vessel, preventing the build-up of plaque, which can lead to heart attack, stroke, and other cardiovascular problems. This makes NO an anti-atherogenic or preventer of clogs.

8. The result is open blood vessels with an increased flow of blood (Cooke, et. al., 2002).

When produced in various parts of the body, NO can cause erection, decrease inflammation, and fight off infection and other immune system problems, e.g. cancerous tumors. Where the nerves spread out into the peripheral areas, NO is utilized to regulate several things, including diverse genitourinary, respiratory, gastrointestinal, and tract functions (Moncada and Higgs, 1993). It is also a neurotransmitter that has some input into memory when utilized in the central nervous system. In fact, NO, acting through cGMP, is part of several important brain functions (Roizen, et. al., 2008). Amazingly, this mighty little molecule did not receive notice for its abilities until fifty years ago.

History

The story of nitric oxide (NO) as beneficial does not begin until the 1980s. Until then, the only mention of NO was in reference to its actions as a component of smog (Butler, et. al., 2003). It was considered a toxic substance that produced harmful results when active in the environment. The rehabilitation of NO began to occur after the 1980 research made by Furchgott and Zadwazki. They published an article on the endothelial cells and what was called the endothelium-derived relaxing factor (EDRF) (Bryan and Murad, 2010). The EDRF was as yet unidentified.

In 1987 and 1988, several British researchers headed by Salvatore Moncada conducted studies of the EDRF. Their findings led them to the conclusion that not only was NO the EDRF, but L-arginine was the enzyme responsible for production of NO (Cooke and Zimmer, 2002). They published their findings in *Nature*. Theirs was a finding that shook the scientific community. Many were unwilling to believe that a substance such as NO, so toxic outside the body, was beneficial within it.

Research continued to amass to support the findings of Moncado and colleagues. This eventually led in 1992 to the declaration by *Science* that nitric oxide was the "Molecule of the Year" (Bryan & Murad, 2010; Fried, et. al., 1999). During that period, publications on NO rose from a paltry few, climbing to eight thousand in 1996 and thirteen thousand in 1997 (Vallance, 1998; Fried, et. al., 1999). By 2002, the number had climbed to approximately fifty-two hundred with one hundred thousand by 2010 (Jugdutt, 2004; Bryan and Loscalzo, 2011).

Highlights of this period include work by Ferid Murad, Robert Furchgott, and Louis J. Ignarro. Collectively and/or separately, they proved NO acted as a signaling device within the cardiovascular system. In other words, it sent a message off resulting in the performance of certain necessary functions. Their discoveries resulted in the awarding of the Nobel Prize for Physiology and Medicine in 1998 (Ignarro, 2000). Yet, for some unknown but often commented on reason, Moncada was not recognized in this fashion, although he has received other prestigious awards.

By the end of the century and into the next, researchers had embarked on a thorough exploration of the role NO plays in the body. They had begun to identify the biological tasks the molecule played to keep balance and proper function. The list is an impressive one (Vallance, 1998). Although tiny in shape, simple in design, and with a small life span, NO is found to play a significant part in the following systems within the body:

- Cardiovascular

- Respiratory

- Host defense

- Nervous

- Musculoskeletal

- Gastrointestinal

- Haemopoietic

- Genitourinary

In the past decades, NO has emerged as one of the most significant molecules. It acts as a biological mediator, playing a major role in processes that embrace everything from neurological functions to the annihilation of pathogens (Thomas, et. al., 2010).

Conclusion

After years of neglect and derision, NO has been declared a hero in the world of human biology. It is now the topic of much research and speculation. Studies are in progress as researchers sort out the effect the release of this simple gas has on the human body and its systems. While debate is ongoing as to the exact amount and such things as benefits and deleterious effects, serious work continues in certain major areas with research branching out into various aspects of NO. Research also looks at the possible applications of NO, including medical. While NO may not be a magic bullet for all persons and their health issues, it has become an important factor in various fields of science. These include sports medicine and nutrition. Medical application has become an increasingly interesting field of study for researchers and doctors alike as they consider the effect a little or a lot of NO can have on the health and welfare of the human body.

The next section will go beyond the chemistry to explore the sources of NO. This includes both those from natural resources and those artificially manufactured. It will also consider the basic applications suggested by the characteristics and capabilities of NO.

3

Basic Sources of Nitric Oxide

NITRIC OXIDE (NO) does not actually appear out of thin air. While it takes two molecules, one of nitrogen and one of oxygen, to form, the body needs to obtain the material required to manufacture the substance. There are two obvious ways: naturally and synthetically. The body, particularly the endothelium, can produce NO by ingesting a natural substance or by being given a manufactured one.

The natural ways to improve your NO production will be discussed in depth in Chapter 6, as will the use of supplements. This section merely provides a brief overview of the basic sources of NO.

Natural Sources

The major catalyst for the creation of NO is L-arginine. It is found in many food groups, including nuts, meat, fish, and beans (Reizen, et. al., 2008). This is a natural occurrence. The process is a simple one. The individual ingests the product containing L-arginine. It enters the body and into the endothelium.

Once in the endothelium, the L-arginine reacts and produces NO and citrulline. The NO then disperses throughout the system or is targeted to a specific area. NO acts as a messenger, directing the actions of other body components or directly acts upon the cell, blood vessel, or tumor. The specific actions it takes are dependent upon the purpose, the amount present in the body, and the interaction between NO and the targeted area.

Another natural source of NO production is exercise. Exercise helps to release NO. This helps your body breathe more easily. NO can then proceed to boost your immune system and reopen any clogged vessels. The duality of NO also comes into play as a result of exercise. Extensive exercise can result in compromising the immune system. As a result, it is essential to replenish the fluids and nutritional intake. L-arginine foods are the positive source for NO in this instance (Barbarich, 2010; Sears, 2010).

As well as food, drink can affect the levels of NO in your body. While shakes and nutritional drinks made from food high in arginine are a good source, there are other options. According to several studies, both wine and chocolate are also positive sources from which to obtain NO (Gresele, Pignatelli, Guglielmini, Carnevale, Mezzasoma, Ghiselli, Momi, and Violi, 2008). The best wine to drink is red (Roizen, et. al., 2008; Maroon, 2009). The only chocolate that results in high levels of NO production is pure dark chocolate or cocoa (Maroon, 2009).

Yet if you are unable to obtain your NO from natural sources, you can turn elsewhere. NO can also be the result of the introduction of other substances, including specific drugs.

NO-Based Drugs—NO-NSAIDs and Others: A Question of Effectiveness

Several drugs now fall into what are termed NO-NSAIDs. These are nitric oxide-based non-steroidal anti-inflammatory drugs. Often called NO donors, these are products currently in the development and testing phases (Dunlap, Abdul-Hay, Chandrasena, Hagos, Sinha, and Wang, 2008). They promise to decrease the side-effects associated with NSAIDs. These are notably an irritation of the stomach lining, which could result in the development of ulcers (Bonavida, Baritaki, Huerta-Yepez, Vega, Jazirehi, and Berenson, 2010).

What is also appealing about the NO-NSAIDs is the lower cost and efficacy of the drugs. This is particularly true in the application as cancer treatment. It combines with excellent results with both chemo and radiotherapy

(Hirst and Robson, 2010). NO is able to sensitize cancer tumors to chemicals and radiotherapy while slowing down their growth.

The advantages of NO-NSAIDs over regular NSAIDs are several and significant. NO-NSAIDs require less dosage to accomplish the same result. NO-NSAIDs have a stronger potency. They are gentler on the system than NSAIDs. NO-NSAIDs are also less toxic. This makes them a cost-effective, safe alternative (Burgund, et. al., 2002; Bonavida, et. al., 2010; Bonavida, 2010).

Among the possible NO-NSAIDs for future use are:

- NO-aspirin

- NO-diclofenac

- NO-naproxen

- NO-ibuprofen

- S-NO-diclofenac

NO Inhalers

One form of regulated and available NO comes in inhalers. This is a carefully controlled and monitored form of NO gas, usually called medical-grade gas. It has been approved for use among infants but not, as yet, for adults. The dosages in both cases are small and produce few if any side effects (Ichinose and Zapol, 2004; Griffiths and Evans, 2005; Bonavida, 2010).

ACTIONS OF NO INHALERS

They release NO into the airways and respiratory system to reduce swelling of the passageways to and in the lungs. Research in both 2002 and 2010 has resulted in several drugs being placed upon the market. The focus has been on the use in Neonatal intensive care units (NICU). NO is inhaled as a means of helping premature babies with respiratory problems breathe easily without any significant side effects (Burgaud, Ongini, and Del Soldato, 2002; Lee, et. al., 2010). An example of this is the common INOmax.

Research indicates the positive use of NO in this situation. A summary of the research by R. Inchose and his co-researchers (2004) provides informative data on the ability of NO to treat hypoxic respiratory problems in infants. The gas is produced and inhaled. Once released into the bloodstream, NO reacts with oxyhemoglobin and deoxyhemoglobin to form other substances. In the process of performing this, NO acts as a very selective pulmonary (related to the lungs) vasodilator (Ichinose, et. al., 2004). It does not direct its energies elsewhere but concentrates on the lungs.

In the case where adults formed the basis of the research, NO released into the bloodstream was less successful. The results demonstrated only partial success. The effects of NO produced and introduced in this fashion proved successful only as a supportive measure in adults suffering from acute hypoxia and hypertension (Griffiths and Evans, 2005). It proved ineffective and/or exhibited short-term positive results in those adult individuals who had acute lung injury or acute respiratory distress syndrome (ARDS). Dosage of NO does seem to play a role in the effectiveness, but further research is required before the mechanisms of both success and failure are completely understood.

Sex, Drugs, and NO

In addition to oral NO-SAIDs and NO inhalers, there are also other ways to take and use your NO. NO drugs have been created to correct sexual dysfunction. These are readily available on the market. Among the most common are sildenafi, vardenafil, and tadalafil, sold as Viagra®, Levitra®, and Cialis®.

The small pill known as Viagra® rocked the world in more ways than one. It became one of the most successful drugs ever launched in history. When it emerged, it created a media sensation, receiving far more press coverage than the discovery of nitric oxide or its role.

Conclusion

NO can occur naturally within the body. It arises out of the body's ingestion of L-arginine. This is common in certain food and drinks. Exercise can also stimulate the production of NO. Too much exercise, however, can cause a depletion of NO in your bloodstream and reduce the ability of your immune system to protect itself from bacteria and viruses.

The source of NO may also be artificially constructed. NO gas may be made according to strict conditions in the laboratory for use in treating certain respiratory problems of infants. Use has yet to be approved for adults, where application seems to be less successful than in infant respiratory problems.

Currently, testing and trials are taking place on the latest form of NO: NO-NSAIDs. The initial results seem promising. This source of NO results in fewer side effects than the current crop of NSAIDs does. Among the possibilities for the treatment of potential medical issues are NO-aspirin and NO-ibuprofen. With a smaller amount and less toxicity, NO-SAIDs can fulfill the same function as the traditional NSAIDs. These are the new sources of NO for the future.

4

Nitric Oxide and Medical Applications

NITRIC OXIDE (NO) has commanded attention within the medical community since it was discovered that it fulfilled several important functions in the human body. Indeed, the possible applications of NO were so many it seemed impossible to believe. Yet as research continued—and continues today—the original findings were merely the tip of the proverbial iceberg.

General Health Benefits of NO

The list of general health benefits attributed to NO and acting within diverse biological systems are impressive (Lee, Kim, Jo, Pae, and Chung, 2010). They are not restricted to one specific body part or system. In fact, due to the size and range of the endothelium, the existence of the tiny molecule NO has the potential to affect a wide variety of significant body systems (Clarke, et. al., 2002). Among the currently noted benefits of the release of NO into the body are:

1. Lowering of blood pressure

2. Improving blood circulation

3. Delaying onset of atherosclerosis (hardening of the arteries)

4. Reducing and even preventing the risk of stroke and/or heart attack

5. Reducing pregnancy-related hypertension

6. Regulation of insulin secretion

7. Controlling the airways to the lung

8. Relaxing your sphincter vessels

9. Ensuring blood flow to the brain

10. Releasing human growth hormone (HGH)

NO is touted as being antimicrobial, anti-inflammatory, and anti-oxidative against various disease states (Lee, et. al., 2010). In other words, the presence of NO within the body helps to fight off disease, reduce swelling, and protect the cells within the body from any harmful effects of oxidation. NO is also a neurotransmitter. Acting as a messenger, it sends signals to other components of the body, including other messengers, to perform a specific task.

Reasons for Poor Endothelium Health

NO is the body's natural defense against many health problems. It is also completely essential. Yet it requires a healthy vehicle to ensure it is able to carry on its tasks. This is the endothelium. The endothelium may not be in good health for several reasons. These may be the result of structural problems such as impairment of or damage to the endothelium itself. This will result in decreased or even a lack of NO production.

Poor endothelium health can also arise from the presence or lack of certain substances. If, for example, there is a lack of NOS (nitric oxide synthase) in the blood vessel wall or insufficient amounts of various cofactors in the process (e.g., tetrahydrobioterin), the endothelium cannot produce sufficient NO. This decreases the health within the endothelium itself and, therefore, affects other systems dependent upon the ongoing release of NO. One particular molecule negatively impacting the health of the endothelium is ADMA. This is found in the blood of those individuals with or at serious risk of heart disease (Thomas, et. al, 2010; Cooke, et. al., 2002).

In essence, anything that prevents the formation of NO is harmful for the endothelium. Whatever the cause of poor endothelium health is also responsible for many detrimental effects upon the human body. A lack of NO due to a dysfunctional endothelium or otherwise can and does over time have serious effects upon the human body (Anker and Eberhardt, 2004). Among the possible results are diabetes mellitus and prinzmetal angina (Jugdutt, 2004). From the beginning, however, studies have focused on the impact of NO on the cardiovascular system.

NO and Cardiovascular Health

Nitric Oxide is absolutely essential for maintaining the health of your cardiovascular system (Esselstyn, 2008). This is the system responsible for many life-continuing actions. NO is a regulator of the blood that flows in and out as well as a preventive measure (Napoli, Crimini, Williams-Ignarro, de Nigris, and Ignarro, 2010). Its overall release into the blood stream results in several positive effects upon the affected components of the cardiovascular system.

WHAT IS THE CARDIOVASCULAR SYSTEM?

The cardiovascular system is composed of the heart, the blood vessels that transport the blood and waste products, and blood (Markovitch, 2006). It is responsible for several important functions within the body. These include:

- The delivery of oxygen (O_2) and amino acids, glucose, and other nutrients to all the tissues of the body

- The transporting of such metabolic waste products as urea (a component of urine) as well as carbon dioxide (CO_2) from the various tissues to the lungs and the excretory organs

- Delivering electrolytes, water, and specific hormones all over the human body

- Making a contribution to the body's immune system

- Regulation of heat and cold to maintain a steady temperature—or thermoregulation (Aaronson and Ward, 2010)

Within this system, each component has its own particular task to carry out. NO works to aid in the performance of these diverse undertakings.

WHAT NO DOES

No acts positively within the blood stream to accomplish a variety of tasks. These include the following:

- Relaxation of the arteries

- Opening of the coronary arteries

- Lowering the serum cholesterol levels

- Preventing the oxidization of so-called "bad" LDL cholesterol

- Acting as a blood thinner or anticoagulant (Fried, et. al., 1999; Cooke, et. al., 2002)

In doing so, NO prevents or reduces the occurrence of more serious cardio-vascular problems such as stroke, angina, heart disease, and heart attack.

HOW NO WORKS

NO works within the endothelium of the blood vessels. Once it is sent into the system through the natural release from L-arginine or other NOS, it acts as a messenger and a vasodilator to create smooth, large, and non-sticky passageways for the blood to course through. By doing this, NO creates a non-sticky surface. Some researchers refer to it as Teflon-like in its ability to prevent any undesirable body from sticking to or clumping within it (Essel-styne, 2008; Fried, et. al., 1999; Cooke, et. al., 2002). As a result, the blood vessels are able to slough off such things as plaque build-up and prevent the clumping together of blood platelets.

NO also helps the blood vessels to relax, which encourages smoother and more rapid blood flow. This action plays an important role in maintaining blood pressure and reducing hypertension or high blood pressure (HBP). The actions of NO also play a role in diminishing or preventing other cardiovas-cular problems. Besides HBP, NO plays a role in controlling atherosclerosis or hardening of the arteries.

If an individual has high blood pressure or hardening of the arteries, health issues occur. These two particular problems result in severe heart problems: heart failure and stroke. Another possible cardiovascular problem that could occur if the arteries are not kept slick and the blood left to flow swiftly is angina. This sense of restriction is the result of the coronary arteries narrowing, restricting blood flow (Jugdutt, 2004). The ability of NO to keep the cardiovascular system free and clear of such impediments as plaque and clots permits the system to function at its optimum level.

FACTORS AFFECTING NO'S ABILITY

Vascular problems such as stroke, high blood pressure, and hardening of the arteries can also possibly be prevented or reduced through the powers of NO. There are, however, certain factors that will affect the ability of NO to help you avoid or restrict these health issues. Among the most common that interfere with the production of NO, many are preventable. These include:

- High cholesterol

- Smoking

- Alcohol

- Prescription drugs

- Fatty foods

- Weight

- Diabetes

- Hypertension

- A sedentary lifestyle

- Stress

All these factors can restrict the production of NO. Fatty foods, for example, reduce the amount of NO production significantly. Smoking actually inhibits the endothelium from producing NO, stopping the process before it can start (Roizen, et. al., 2008). Stress is also a preventive measure against your body's manufacturing and retaining the right amount of NO.

Smoking and diet are two major factors that are significant contributors to poor NO production. As noted previously, research does indicate the blocking of the manufacture of NO by fatty foods. This results in the clogging up of the arteries by substances to create plaque. The result affects the ability of the cardiovascular system to function properly.

Research into smoking indicates the negative effects this habit has on both the endothelial cells and the production of NO. Cigarette smoking exerts influence on both the endothelial cells and the production of NO. The ability of NO to result in the vasodilation (widening) of the arteries is severely impaired. The enzyme responsible to derive NO—the endothelium (e) NOS—decreases its activity (Su, Han, Giraldo, and Black, 1998). In the process, smoking affects the coronary arteries in terms of elasticity and structure. This is related to the decrease in the availability of NO (Guo, Oldham, Kelienman, Phalen, and Hassab, 2006).

The lack of NO in smokers' systems is said to account for their high risk of cardiovascular and pulmonary disease (Su, et. al., 1998). Stopping smoking gives your endothelium the chance to repair its own cellular damage. It can then produce the right amount of NO for the body's needs. This is only possible, however, if smoking has continued only for a short time. In the case of long-term smokers, the damage to the arteries is irreversible (Guo, et. al., 2006).

As a result of smoking, problems emerging in your cardiovascular, digestive, respiratory, immune, and endocrine systems find a foothold and/or increase substantially. You place yourself at greater risk for those diseases and health issues. They are opportunists that can gain a toehold and spread because NO is unavailable or is only available in too small amounts.

You can prevent this from happening by stopping these practices and/or getting control over the medical or physical problem. Reduce your hypertension. Lose weight. Watch what you eat. Stop smoking and get out and exercise. This will ensure you have fewer health problems, increase your body's ability to manufacture NO, and help the endothelium in its fight to restore the ability of NO to fight back (Sears and Sears, 2010). Many health problems can be reversed if you reverse the causal factor and reintroduce the right amounts of NO back into the systems.

There are also, however, factors affecting NO that you can do little if anything about. Your genetics will dictate certain aspects of your body composition and how it both acts and reacts. Another factor over which you have no control is your age. The levels of NO within the body decline as you grow older. Some differences between the decrease of NO production and gender exist. Levels are higher for women than men. This bias dissipates soon after women reach menopause. Postmenopausal levels of women are equal to those found in men.

NO and Your Immune System

NO plays an important part in helping your immune system to combat diseases. NO responds in a way that acts to protect your body and help maintain it in good health.

WHAT IS THE IMMUNE SYSTEM?

The immune system comprises various different components working throughout your body to destroy diseases and prevent the invasion of disease-causing bacteria (Markovitch, 2006). One small fighter in this life-long battle for the body's health is the macrophage, a type of white cell. These tiny organisms seek out and destroy all incoming invaders. They are scavengers on a singular mission. In addition to destruction, they also act as messengers, telling other parts of the system what to do, whom to attack, and when and where to mobilize. Other components of the army that makes up the immune system are T-cells, B-cells, thymus, bone marrow, the spleen, and lymphatic system (Roizen and Mehmet, 2005).

The role of the immune system, overall, is to fight off any foreign invaders. To do so, it relies on aggressive toxic agents such as nitric oxide (Butler, et. al, 2003).

ACTIONS AND EFFECT OF NO ON THE IMMUNE SYSTEM

NO has been considered a mediator of acute inflammation (Tierney, McPhee, and Papadakis, 2006). It has also been considered a vasodilator. As a result, NO, along with other free radicals, regulates the immune response. This includes roles in:

- Vasodilation

- Bronchodilation

- Neurotransmission

- Tumor surveillance

- Anti-microbial defenses (Lee, et. al., 2010; Esselstyn, 2008)

NO adopts any and all of these roles within the immune system.

In the immune system, NO is activated in the cells by cytokines (small proteins). It is then the job of NO to act as a destroyer of the invaders. Macrophages also produce the same result. They release NO, which acts as a toxic agent (Marcovitch, 2006). NO proceeds to attack and kill all foreign bacteria and viruses. This also includes cancerous tumors (Fried, et. al., 1999).

NO AND CANCER

Perhaps where the study of NO has offered great promise is in its ability to inhibit the growth of cancer tumor cells. NO, as part of an active immune system, is able to slow down the growth of these cells (Bonavida, 2010). Research indicates that NO can be both a vasodilator and cause apoptosis or death of a cell. Both can prove beneficial in helping the immune system defend itself against cancerous growths. If used at the right dosage, NO can be absolutely toxic to tumor cells (Butler, et. al, 2003). This is one possible situation when NO-NSAIDS (nitric oxide non-steroidal anti-inflammatory drugs) may prove beneficial (Bonavida, 2010). Further research needs to establish specific dosages and how NO can be used to benefit sufferers of this deadly disease.

NO also acts as a warning of problems. If the levels of NOS2 are high, it is indicative the cancer is of a type with a poor survival rate (Cheng, Ridnow, Glynn, Switzer, Flores-Santana, Hussain, Thomas, Ambs, Harris, and Wink, 2010). The only exception is noticeable in the cases of lung and ovarian cancer.

NO IN ACTION AGAINST CANCER CELLS

When enzymes, proteins of other members of the immune system, attack cells, they tend to be restricted to one of two basic methods: necrosis or apoptosis. With necrosis, the less than subtle destruction of a cell, NO uses a direct and heavy approach, one akin to what Butler (2003) calls a sledge hammer. With apoptosis, death of a cell is slow, very controlled, and orchestrated. It is death through planning. It is rare for a molecule to be involved in both types of cell destruction. NO, again, defies the mode.

Where NO excels in the treatment of cancer is its ability to mimic individual treatments and cancer foes. It not only acts like other inhibitors of metastasis (malignant growth process), but also acts like anti-angiogenic drugs, therefore inhibiting the growth of blood vessels (Hirst, et. al., 2010; Bonavida, et. al., 2010).

The efficacy of NO has also been found to increase when it has been used in combination with other cancer therapies. This is particularly true when NO is combined with chemotherapy or radiotherapy (Hirst, et. al., 2010). In fact, NO can help sensitize tumor growths, making them more vulnerable to such therapy.

NO is truly a powerful weapon the body uses in the battle to defeat all invaders, including any cancerous growth. If the body lacks the ability to produce NO, or if the amounts of NO are insufficient, immune deficiency is a serious possibility (Jugdutt, 2004).

THE OTHER SIDE OF NO

While this is actually a topic for the final chapter, it needs to be mentioned here. Although NO can reduce and destroy cancer cells, it can also promote them. The factors, still under consideration in research, are:

- The concentration of NO in the tissues

- The sources of the NO

- The existence of reactive molecules

Such factors will affect whether NO is going to promote or destroy cancer within the human body (Garbán, 2010).

Addressing Respiratory Problems

Everyone needs to breathe. Failure to do so leads to comas, failure of the body to function, and death. NO plays a significant role in helping you breathe. Without it, the respiratory system would be unable to function as effectively as its needs to.

WHAT IS THE RESPIRATORY SYSTEM?

According to *Black's Medical Dictionary* (Markovitch, 2006), the respiratory system consists of all the organs and any of the tissues that are associated with breathing (respiration). This includes your nose (nasal cavity), throat (pharynx), voice box (larynx), trachea, bronchi, and lungs. All play an important role in ensuring you are able to breathe in oxygen and breathe out carbon dioxide. NO plays an important function in ensuring you continue to take in air.

WHAT NO DOES

Research on the use of NO as a drug to abet respiratory problems is still in its infancy. Preliminary research is promising for children, if not adults. Nevertheless, if someone has suffered from smoke inhalation, NO is considered beneficial since it helps to reduce any acute inflammation responsible for difficulty in breathing.

According to some studies, NO has an indirect impact on the airways of the lung. It not only lets you breathe easier but also helps to prevent the onset of various common lung problems (Fried, et. al., 1999). Research indicates that newborn babies with respiratory failure improve considerably when given NO to inhale (Butler, et. al, 2003).

The inhalers are one of several new NSAIDs. The version applied to infants born prematurely in the neonatal critical care units are referred to as NO-NSAIDs—nitric oxide NSAIDs (Bonavida, 2010). The NO, once breathed in, works to relax the smooth muscles that comprise the lungs. They, therefore, dilate the lung's blood vessels and allow for the free passage of both air/oxygen and blood. What is also promising is the lack of any severe or even serious side effects. Research indicates that temporary raspy breathing is the major indicator of and basic side effect stemming from the use of a NO-NSAID.

Endocrine Glands

The human body consists of many vitally important parts. Among the most important is the complex system of organs called the endocrine glands or endocrine system.

WHAT ARE THE ENDOCRINE GLANDS OR ENDOCRINE SYSTEM?

The two terms—endocrine glands and endocrine system—are often interchangeable (Markovitch, 2006). The endocrine glands are responsible for producing hormones that direct the body to start, speed up, slow down, and even cease certain actions. Among the glands related to NO activities are the adrenal glands, the pancreas, and the hypothalamus.

This important system acts as a control center or system for the entire body. The glands are found in separate areas of the body. Among the more important glands involved in the processes of NO are the hypothalamus, the adrenals, and the pancreas. Important organs include the liver, the gonads, the kidneys, and the heart.

The endocrine glands consist of four major components to be considered here:

1. The hypothalamus—This is located in the forebrain. Its main purpose is to perform as a thermo-regulator or body temperature controller.

2. The pancreas—The pancreas is found just below the stomach. The pancreatic duct attaches this organ to the small intestine. Two hormones originate in this gland: insulin and glucagon. Both act to control blood sugar levels. If one or the other becomes imbalanced, the results can be dangerous and even fatal.

3. The adrenal medulla—Located just above the kidney, the adrenal glands number two and are responsible for the production of adrenaline and noradrenaline. These two hormones aid with the constriction of the blood vessels in two distinct areas: the skin and the abdomen (barring the intestines).

4. Gonads: These are sex glands. They are either the testes or ovaries.

Within the endocrine system, certain glands send signals or chemical messages to other parts of the human body. They tell the specific component to enable the action of certain functions. Hormones can also speed up the process and slow it down.

WHAT DOES NO DO?

NO definitely has an impact on or influence over the endocrine system. The pancreas is responsible for the production of insulin. NO can help regulate insulin fabrication. In helping the pancreas keep the process of insulin production and release under control, NO can actually decrease the risk of an individual's becoming diabetic.

NO also acts within the adrenal glands. Its purpose here is to ensure the release of the hormone adrenaline. Andrenaline is the "flight-or-fight" response. It comes into play in a variety of scenarios. Adrenaline is also a necessary element of ensuring the body can perform at its peak during exercise and in competitive events.

In regards to the sex glands, NO has a specific function. The release of gonadotropin hormones is also a property of NO. As a result, NO helps the body to define what is physically female and male. In literature and advertisements for bodybuilding, this result is touted as a manliness factor. It becomes part of the selling point of supplements that contain the NO-producing L-arginine. Such ads fail to mention that NO is not species specific and that gonadotrophin refers to the hormone that stimulates both male and female sex organs to secrete testosterone and estrogen (Rushton, 2004).

The Brain and the Central Nervous System

While, arguably, some NO functions are related to the hypothalamus—located in the brain—some are distinct in their relationship with the brain. NO acts within the structure referred to as the central nervous system to help in the neurotransmission of certain actions.

WHAT IS THE CENTRAL NERVOUS SYSTEM?

The central nervous system (CNS) is home to several significant body organs, nerve cells, and body parts. In particular, it is where you will find the spinal cord and the brain (Markovitch, 2006). The brain is the control center of the entire body. From its position, it sends off and receives messages. Every day, it works to control such things as:

- Breathing

- Thought processes

- Body temperature

- Sensations such as seeing, feeling, hearing

- Speech

- Heart beat

Yet the brain, like the rest of the body, depends upon certain enzymes, proteins, and other related matter to help it accomplish these tasks. One of the helpers in several tasks is NO.

NO IN THE BRAIN

Researchers have located three types of NOS—the enzymes that help produce NO from L-arginine—in the brain. All perform specific tasks. There is only one problem. Science is still working out which functions and the extent of their influence the various NOS perform (Butler, et. al., 2003).

1. iNOS—related to the immune system. It is found in the glial cells. What it does is not yet known.

2. nNOS—referring to the nervous system. It is in the nerve cells (neurons). It helps in the learning process.

3. eNOS—indicating endothelium origins. They perform the same function in all endothelial cells: enlarge and keep them free of any flotsam and jetsam.

What NO Does

The brain is the home of all three types of NOS producing NO molecules for specific purposes within the central nervous system. NO is, nevertheless, derived from the amino acid arginine. For example, in the brain, argentine-derived NO is responsible for orchestrating the flow of blood (Fried, et. al., 1996).

Yet the NO molecules do not act alone. In the brain, NO uses cGMP (short for cyclic guanosine monophosphate) to accomplish what it needs to do. In the process, cGMP acts as a second messenger, not the original signaler. NO has one property that helps it accomplish its tasks. The gas easily crosses the cell membranes to bind directly to guanylyl cyclose.

The relationship between NO and the brain is diverse, a word commonly applied to the functions of NO. NO can alter the computational ability to calculate that is part of brain function (*Science Daily*, 2008). The molecule also acts in other important functions. Among these is memory (Butler, et. al, 2003).

The exact function of NO in the learning process is not yet mapped. It does help individuals understand and learn. It is particularly noted for the function called long-term memory. Researchers have remarked upon the need for NO in the brain for this feature to work properly. It is also speculated that one of the contributing causes to such problems as Parkinson's disease and Alzheimer's is the effect that inadequate production of NO has on the brain (Butler, et. al, 2003; Fried, et. al., 1999).

NO is also considered to be a neurotransmitter. In the brain, the most common ones are dopamine, serotonin, and endorphins. The actions of NO, however, are somewhat different than the traditional type. NO behaves in a less restricted fashion. It crosses barriers. Nevertheless, it is released into the post-synaptic nerve to carry out its message.

A summary of NO's functions in the brain would have to include the following:

- Brain blood flow

- Promotion of angiogenesis

- Maintenance of a cellular redox state

- Cell immunity

- Neuronal survival

Research and scientific speculation also indicate several other roles for NO. The ability of the adult brain to be flexible is due to NO. Research has also indicated that in individuals suffering from a stroke, an increased production of NO can decrease the chances of brain damage when compared to those who did not have it (Sears, et. al., 2010).

NO and the Digestive System

Your digestive system, including your stomach, is not unaffected by the release of NO. NO plays a significant role in what is termed the gastrointestinal tract of the body.

WHAT IS THE GASTROINTESTINAL TRACT?

The gastrointestinal tract (GI) is the components of the body that handle your digestion of nutrients and elimination of waste (Markovitch, 2006). It is one of the largest systems in your body. The GI tract consists of the following, listed from the top down:

- Mouth

- Throat (pharynx)

- Oesophagus or gullet

- Stomach

- Small intestine, consisting of twenty-two feet (five to six meters), on average, of tubing

- Large intestine—wider than the small intestine but only six feet (one to eight meters) in length

- Colon—another name for the large intestine

- Rectum—the exit point

When considering the part acted by NO, research looks at its relationship to the various functions of the stomach.

NO AND THE STOMACH

The behavior of NO within the GI tract and the stomach in particular has resulted in mixed reports. When taken in some types of supplements, particularly those involved in the sport of bodybuilding, it may result in stomach upset. It can give you cramps, nausea, and other unpleasant symptoms. Whether this is the result of the specific formulation, the delivery system, or the levels of NO introduced into the system has as of yet not been explored in the research.

This actually contradicts what NO can and does accomplish in its healing capacity within the stomach. During the 1990s, a significant amount of research focused on the effect of the release of NO into the stomach or gut. The conclusions considered the ability of NO to act in two capacities:

- As a relaxer of the stomach lining

- Protector of the stomach and its lining

Swedish researchers found data supporting the positive aspects of NO in both capacities. It did perform as a relaxing factor (MacNaughton, Wallace, Cirino, and Wallace, 1989). NO also acted as a defense against acidic digestive juices (*Reader's Digest*, 2010; McNaughton, et. al., 1989). The release of nitric oxide was found to lessen the formation, continuation, and pain of stomach ulcers (Desai, Sessa, and Vane, 1991).

Erectile Dysfunction

Researchers have begun to explore the application of NO in different ways. The discovery of the molecule has resulted in several novel ways of treating patients with a variety of different problems. Among the most touted is the use of NO to decrease the problem of erectile dysfunction. When researchers noted that NO was able to enlarge the blood vessels, it set some scientists off into exploring a practical application. The result was, among others, sildenafil or Viagra® (Fried, et. al., 1999; Butler, et. al, 2003). This is a drug utilizing NO in its role as a vasodilator. The logic is as follows:

1. The penis consists of blood vessels.

2. When the blood vessels engorge, the penis swells and becomes active.

3. NO can accomplish this if it is positioned correctly.

4. A drug using NO or a similar substance could create this scenario.

The result was the creation of several drugs, including sildenafil, vardenafil, and tadalafil. All work on the basic principle that if NO is discharged within the body from the endings of the nerves closest to the penile blood vessels (nervi erigentes), it will activate the guanylyl cyclase and produce cyclic guanosine monophosphate or cGMP. cGMP is a very powerful vasodilator and will cause the blood to flow to the penis. This will result in an erection.

The process is not actually simple. It is related to the possible involvement of each, one, or even all of the three NOS enzymes. The overall result from initial stimulus or stimuli involves several neurotransmitters. It ends up being a cascade effect with each step needing to be successful if the final action is to take place (Butler, et. al., 2003).

Sildenafil caused a sensation. It was the first time the discovery of a pill based on scientific knowledge had received such media attention. This ranged from notice in the scientific press to bad jokes and puns on late-night talk shows. In the mainstream reports, little to no mention was made of the role of NO.

Yet all is not right within the "NO produces working sex function" equation. While providing NO to the body does help with this serious medical problem, it can create issues. Research indicates that NO is also implicated in sexual dysfunction. It can result specifically in male infertility as a result of a too-low sperm count (European Society for Human Reproduction and Embryology, 2006). It seems too-high levels of NO are the culprit.

NO for "Female Problems"

Besides treating sexual problems in the male, NO can be applied to those affecting women. NO engorges the female genetalia in a fashion similar to how it affects the male penis (Roizen, et. al., 2008). There is a partial truth concerning the production of NO, eating L-arginine, and sexual arousal. According to one theory, if women entering menopause eat foods high in L-arginine, they will increase their desire/libido. Since a decreased sex drive is one of the "downers" of entering menopause, this may come as a relief to many women and their partners.

What Is This about NO and Longevity?

According to some research, NO is capable of reducing the effects of the passage of time. NO releases the growth hormone known as HGH (human growth hormone). This is the so-called "key" to a long life (Fried, et. al., 1999). NO is also involved in many of the important functions of the body that alter as we get old. In fact, the production is also affected by the onset of age. It decreases. While, until after menopause, women are less affected than men, both genders experience age-related NO loss. This leads to the speculation that if NO production were maintained at certain levels, the signs or at least many of the physiological aspects of aging may decrease. Certain researchers and medical professionals support this theory. Among them are Joseph Maroon (2009), Louis Ignarro, and William Sears (Sears, et. al, 2010).

The evidence used to support this theory is based on several perceptions and understandings about the chemistry and functions of NO within the body. In part it relates to the ability of NO to widen the blood vessels and arteries. Another factor affecting the ongoing belief in a cure for the aging process is the decrease in NO production as humans age.

A number of physiological changes occur when people age. Among them are several that are related to NO functions. Aging affects the heart muscle. It becomes stiffer while the blood vessels tend to narrow. NO controls the enlarging of the blood vessels. If there is too little, hardening of the arteries and clogging of blood vessels occur.

During the aging process, the lungs become stiff and the air passageways become narrow. This decreases the intake of oxygen. It is a function of NO to widen the airway passages. In doing so, it makes breathing easier.

Other changes that involve a decrease in the amount of NO manufactured include a dysfunctional sex drive, weakening of the immune system, mood disorders, and several endocrine-related problems such as diabetes mellitus, high blood pressure, and high cholesterol (Sears, et. al., 2010). The loss of the elasticity or tone of the skin has also been connected to the decrease of NO by some researchers. When NO opens and dilates the arteries beneath the skin, it increases its flexibility. This decreases the depth and amount of wrinkles (Roizen, et. al., 2008).

HOW TO LIVE A LONG, HEALTHY LIFE THROUGH NO

Living longer and healthier has long been the goal of humans. Cortez sough the Fountain of Youth. Other individuals tried to find Shangri-La. For some, while NO may not let you live forever, it can help you delay, slow down, or even prevent some of the negative physical aspects associated with old age.

If you want to keep your body at its prime then NO can offer you some support. It is part of an approach that urges you to become in tune with your body. It is also one that relies on your understanding the body's ability to heal itself. It is a method that requires you to do what is good for your body. This includes eating food that is good for you and, preferably, high in arginine.

If you eat foods that are loaded with L-arginine, you can then increase the levels of NO production. When you do this, you will affect all aspects of your body. In increasing the NO content, you are saying "no" to the deleterious effects of old age. By producing more NO, you encourage and help your body to:

- Have wide arteries and smooth vessel walls, resulting in a strong and healthy heart.

- Keep those airway passages clear and oxygen moving swiftly and freely throughout your body. It will help you breathe easier, avoid respiratory problems and increase your energy level.

- Maintain a healthy sex life.

- Reduce your chances of infections and illnesses. Your immune system will remain strong and capable of fighting against the invaders.

- Retain stable levels of hormones, including insulin. You can reduce the risk of diabetes, HBP, and high blood cholesterol.

According to some perspectives, NO will allow you to have smoother skin and less wrinkles. The flow of blood through the vessels created by NO affects smooth muscle tone and the exterior surface: the skin (Sears, et. al., 2010; Cooke, et. al., 2003; Fried, et. al., 199; Esselstyn, 2008).

This is the miracle of NO. Its multi-tasking and pervasive existence in the human body allows greater scope for hypothesis. While there is some veracity in the ability of NO to help improve life, there is no absolute proof it will actually prolong your life. NO is not the only molecule at work within your body. Furthermore, NO does not work alone. It requires the participation of the rest of the body as host, signaler, means of conveyance, or related functions. There is also one more issue concerning NO to discuss in this chapter, one that can be seen to partially support this theory. What happens when NO fails to function or is dysfunctional?

When NO Fails to Function

It is easy to understand why NO is studied seriously. Its ability to perform so many different roles within the body makes it critical that we understand the extent of its capabilities. Nothing is more capable of making the significance of NO obvious than when research reveals clearly what happens when NO fails to function or functions improperly. At that point, the question arises as to what is not affected by the inability of NO to function or function properly.

According to past and present research, the results are disastrous, if not fatal. A lack of NO has been implicated in the onset and/or growth of several diseases and medical disorders (Anker, et. al., 2004; Bryan, et. al, 2011; Butler, et. al, 2003; Ignarro, 2008). These include increased risks of the following:

- Cancer

- Heart disease

- Heart attack and stroke

- Diabetes mellitus

- Hemorrhoids

- Anal fissures

- Common lung disorders such as coughs, colds, bronchitis

- Tumor growths not all associated with cancer

- Angina

- Atherosclerosis/hardening of the arteries

- High blood pressure/hypertension

- Blood clots and plaque build-up

- Cystic fibrosis

- Infertility

This is just a small list of possibilities, if not probabilities. This chapter has made blatantly clear the widespread impact NO has upon various systems within the body, including both the immune and cardiovascular systems. For example, research has revealed that approximately 95 percent of those suffering from high blood pressure (HBP) have blood vessels that are too stiff to operate correctly (Sears, et. al., 2010). This comes from having too little NO operating within the system. Cancer growths and weakened immune systems are all clear evidence of a malfunctioning endothelial system and/or a deficient amount of NO production. The impact is severe and can ripple throughout the entire body. As a result, when nitric oxide fails to operate or malfunctions, many diverse and serious health problems can occur.

Whither NO

Sex, intellect, the heart, and the lungs—is there anything NO is not involved with? Yet the list above merely scratches the surface. NO research continues to examine where NO acts, interacts, reacts, and overacts or overreacts. In addition to the above-mentioned medical applications and involvement of NO, there are others. NO plays a role in ensuring you have healthy bones and joints. A messenger molecule, it helps with the process of bone resorption or bone destruction (Butler, et. al, 2003). This is part of a natural process if followed by bone deposition (the creation of new bones).

A glance at the literature covering NO research and popular works on the subject provide an inkling of the extent of NO's involvement or possible involvement. A list of topics looks at such things as:

- NO and nerves

- NO and the skin

- NO and vascular cells

- NO and breathing

- NO and exercise

- NO and sports

- NO and waist size

- NO and omega-3

- NO and salmonella bacteria

- NO and the peripheral nervous system

- NO and the central nervous system

- NO and the gastrointestinal system

- NO and bodybuilding

- No and osteoarthritis

It is a vast list and growing. It will continue to expand as researchers discover and hope to learn more about this small molecule.

Conclusion

NO is an almost omnipresent molecule within the human body. It is essential for the proper operation of many functions taken for granted. Without the correct amount directed to the right place, disease and other physical manifestations of health problems will occur. It is for these reasons that it is essential for research to continue to explore this tiny molecule.

As time continues, further studies will illuminate more uses and clarify the application of NO within the context of medicine. Yet even to date, without the benefit of total comprehension of what NO does, the implications and applications are impressive.

5

Nitric Oxide, Exercise, And Sport

WHETHER YOU ARE a professional or amateur athlete, whether you engage in bodybuilding or run marathons, whether you perform yoga movements every day or only take long walks on a weekend, you need to understand the power and purpose of NO and its effect on your ability to exercise and/or take part in sports.

Exercise

Whatever the level of your sporting involvement, exercise keeps you in shape physically and helps you remain mentally active. The benefits of exercise are indeed extensive. While caveats remain based on age, ability, and physical condition, exercise is considered essential by medical professionals and trainers alike.

BENEFITS OF EXERCISE AND NO PRODUCTION

Exercise increases the output of the heart and redistributes blood flow. The result is that more blood flows in the skeletal muscle and circulates in the system. When your body does this, it successfully increases the delivery of oxygen. In turn, this supports further production of breathable air to help continue the exercise response (Shen, Zhang, Zhao, Walin, Sessa, and Hintze, 1995). NO's role in this is to regulate the vascular tone. It accomplishes this by its role as a vasodilator or expander of the blood vessels (Maiorana, O'Driscoll, Taylor, and Green, 2003). It may also be responsible for other as yet certified actions (Shen, et. al., 1995).

Exercise is particularly effective if it is not sporadic. If you want to derive the most from endothelium-derived, exercise-released NO, you need to exercise regularly. While it is believed NO is released during small bouts of exercise such as walking, it is more effective and constant if, like an athlete, you perform on a daily basis over a period of weeks and/or months. This will not only increase your regular production of NO but also regulate it (Maiorana, O'Driscoll, Taylor, and Green, 2003).

The use of exercise on NO may also combine with what is termed a genetic disposition. In other words, an individual who has an innate or natural ability to excel in sports may be able to produce greater amounts of NO through exercising (Shen, et. al.1995). Such a category may include professional athletes and others involved in sports and sporting activities.

WHAT TYPES OF EXERCISE RELEASE NO?

It does not seem to matter which type of exercise you are involved in. Treadmills and elliptical trainers are good examples of a cardiovascular workout in a gym-like and controlled environment. The same benefits can be derived by walking, hiking, trekking, and running. In summer time, swimming, surfing, and boarding are all excellent ways to help you exercise and, therefore, increase the levels and efficiency of NO production. During the winter, you can move the workout indoors and swim in a pool. You can also try snow-shoeing, snowboarding, and/or skiing, both downhill and cross-country.

Exercise fulfills so many different needs of the body. In trying to manufacture more NO, you can reduce your waist size, improve your fitness, and begin to feel more energetic. You will be able to breathe easier with NO working away to keep the blood vessels, arteries, and airways of the heart and lungs clear. Yet, in exercise, as in all aspects of life, you need to be responsible. You need to do what is best for your overall health. If you over-exercise, it may not bring about the desired result of NO production and utilization.

TOO MUCH EXERCISE AND ITS EFFECTS

While NO is released during exercise, it also appears to be depleted if the demands made upon it are too heavy. Consider long-distance runners. After completing a competition, a marathon, or even a strenuous and lengthy training session, the body exhibits not only fatigue but also clinical signs of a decrease in its immune system. This can last from as few as three hours to as long as three days (Barbarich, 2010). If you have a weakened or comprised immune system, you leave yourself open to various illnesses and disease.

Other forms of strenuous activity, including other sports and exercise, can produce identical results. Fortunately, you can replenish your supply of NO and, therefore, help restore the viability of your immune system. You can approach this in several ways. The most common focus is on diet. This includes drinking and eating foods that are high in arginine. Once arginine enters your endothelial cells, it will produce the necessary NO required to do the jobs. At the same time, it will help restore your energy.

Supplements will also provide the necessary NO-producing arginine. Be careful, however. The supplement may actually be counterproductive in certain circumstances.

NO Production and Sports

The role of NO in improving athletic performance is in its infancy in a variety of sport and sport-related activities. Many athletes as yet are not completely aware of the impact of this small molecular gas on the body. The research indicates that specific training regimes can help release and increase NO production in the endothelial cells (Mairoana, et. al., 2003). Furthermore, one of the basic and even essential requirements of sports is energy. If you do not have enough energy, you cannot complete an everyday task, let alone compete.

HOW NO HELPS

NO helps achieve increased levels of energy and aids in improved performance in at least two distinct ways. Opening up the airways of the lungs as well as the blood vessels is part of the basic job description of endothelium-derived NO. These actions allow you to breathe easier and your blood to flow freely. NO production also stimulates the release of hormones in the adrenal glands. This provides you with the adrenaline to respond to the demands of such things as races (Roizen, et. al., 2008). Without the energy provided through the power of NO, athletes would not be able to excel.

One other characteristic drawing attention to this molecule is the role NO plays in the immune system. It is particularly adept at helping with the decrease of inflammation. For athletes of all types, this can help with overcoming minor injuries more quickly. For bodybuilders, this means they can activate NO to reduce the pain resulting from putting their muscles through extremely stressful exercises and positions.

NO is beneficial in this manner, helping in the reduction of inflammation of various sore and painful body parts. Yet you should never rely on it or use it instead of other healing practices. While NO can help reduce oxidative stress and lower the inflammation, rest and the reduction or stopping of such things as exercise and training are also part of repairing your body. NO may accomplish a "quick fix." It will aid in making you feel better, but this does not mean the cause of the symptoms has been adequately addressed. NO is a tool and an aid, not the ultimate answer where physical injury in sport and exercise is concerned. If you want to heal completely and not simply "push through" the injury or pain, talk to a medical professional. Perhaps you can turn to someone in the field of sports medicine for advice. They can help you discover whether increasing NO is the answer or merely a temporary bandage. In consulting a doctor, you are ensuring that the injury is not continued through the misuse of NO.

NO AND BODYBUILDING

While NO production may be of interest to various participants in sports, where it has gained a lot of attention in recent years is in the arena of bodybuilding. The purpose of this competitive and even cut-throat sport is to build up the muscles and increase strength. NO, with its ability to increase the flow of the blood, helps serve this purpose. It is capable of providing the body with faster service of nutrients, particularly to the skeletal muscle structure. In doing so, it helps bodybuilders increase muscle size when they apply stress.

The actions of NO in the immune system are considered helpful in repairing any damage caused by stress during the training.

One further trait that finds favor with bodybuilders is NO's part in the release of hormones. NO acts with the adrenal glands to release the powerful hormone adrenaline. This goes rushing through the system, making anything seem possible—including the lifting of very heavy weights. For runners, this supplies them with that extra energy they need to perform faster.

Bodybuilders do pay careful attention to what they eat. Yet in order to achieve that perfect body, that sculpted form, and ideal body mass, they often turn to other methods that will speed up the process, such as anabolic steroids. All-natural bodybuilders and those who are aware of the serious side effects of steroid use have another option. These are NO supplements. In fact, the passion for bodybuilding has resulted in what can be termed as NO going mainstream.

THE COMMERCIALIZATION OF NO

NO has become part of glitzy and sledgehammer-type advertising campaigns. If you look in any bodybuilding magazine or type the term "nitric oxide" into a search engine, a plethora of articles and advertisements come up. Almost all promote the various miracle-like powers of NO to make your body into an amazing, pumped-up powerhouse. The key words used to sell NO to the public—some who are looking for any means to increase their body mass, become more manly, and improve their strength—are:

- Transformation

- Strength

- Endurance

- Recuperation

- Increased muscle size

- Maleness

- Lean mass gains

- Muscular physique

Everything NO is purported to do as reported in these ads is emphasized using hyperbole and superlatives. NO is not described as a minor player and it certainly does not appear that way in the various paper and electronic media ads. NO is a major component of selling a change in how the individual perceives or wants to actually see his- or herself. The adjectives say it all:

- Muscular

- Lean

- Pumped

- Ripped

- Extreme

- Energized

- Fast

- Massive

- Brutal

- Killer

Consider the article "6 Vein-popping Reasons to Use Nitric Oxide Supplements" (Clark, 2010). This, and other articles on the same site and/or appearing throughout the Net, extol NO supplements as being able to:

- Increase the recovery rate from your gym workouts. Instead of days, the time to recover will be reduced to an unspecified time.

- Reduce that overall sensation of fatigue by boosting your energy levels.

- Enhance your ability to perform long-distance events. Although more applicable to those entered into such things as marathon races or extended track-and-field events, it does appear to be a selling point.

- Energy is more available for your needs.

- Metabolization and use of glucose within the system is increased. In other words, NO acts to help you burn off those extra calories.

- Amplifies that "pumped-up look." The flow of blood to the muscles resulting from triggering NO in the endothelium cells as well as the physical exercise of weight lifting will create the sense of tighter muscles.

While there is some truth, even backed by credible science, behind the claims, do not forget that old Roman saying: "Caveat emptor" or "Let the buyer beware." It is more than applicable.

In the case of NO and NO supplements, the purpose of the various ads says it all. While they make NO appear to be a magic elixir, any result you may obtain is not going to be immediate. While taking NO may have an almost immediate effect on improving your breathing, heart action, and immune system, this does not apply to your musculature. The progression and/or development of your body toward becoming that of the stereotypical body-builder is not guaranteed. It is also not a natural extension of your using NO.

If you are looking for a quick fix to sculpt the perfect body, to appear like the model on the cover of *Muscular Development Magazine*, *Muscle and Fitness*, or *Flex Magazine*, NO is definitely not the answer. This is applicable whether NO enters your body as a part of your diet or in so-called nutritional supplements. Even the most pro-NO ad campaign is wise enough not to promise or make guarantees that this will positively occur.

Companies and retailers know, and you should also realize, that NO supplements may not be suitable for everyone. Those who enter the field of bodybuilding are also smart enough to understand that other factors play an important part in the sport. These include dedication to the regime of the sport. The result should always be careful consideration before you decide to take a nutritional supplement with or without NO.

Factors to Consider When Taking NO Supplements

You need to take precautions if you decide supplements are necessary. Before purchasing any product containing L-arginine—the producer of

NO—talk to a specialist in nutrition as well as someone in the sports field. Do not simply take the word of a supplier, the advertisers, or even a specialized retail outlet or personal trainer.

One reason you need to take precautions concerns regulation. There are currently no regulations on the amount of arginine used in supplements. This means no two NO supplements are alike. It also may cause varied results from taking the purportedly same substance in the same amounts over the same period of time.

What you also need to remember are other factors that can effect the production of NO. You need to look at certain other personal factors that can affect the production of NO within your body as well as the amount you need to take to accomplish your goal. These include:

- Your age: NO production decreases as you age. This will affect the dosage you may need to take to reach your stated goals.

- Your gender: Women produce more NO than men until they reach menopause. This will help you determine how much of the supplement you will require.

- Your health and medical record: If you are suffering from serious health conditions, do NOT take NO supplements without consulting your medical professional. The supplements, which consist of a variety of substances besides arginine, may produce negative side effects that can imperil your health. The relationship between the levels of NO in your system and the result in either positive or negative effects is a complex one. Talk to a professional before you make your decision.

- Consider your current diet: Will taking the supplements increase the levels too high, have adverse effects, or disrupt the balance of your overall system?

- One other factor to consider if you are female is pregnancy. It is never recommended that women who are pregnant take NO supplements. It can be harmful to both your body and that of the unborn child.

- Women should also not take arginine supplements if they are lactating.

- If lack the motivation or dedication to follow through with an entire system that utilizes NO as part but not all of it.

Look carefully over these important aspects of your lifestyle. Also consider other things such as any other medication or supplements you are taking. This includes herbal products. Medical practitioners have become aware that herbal supplements and other forms of medicine may not only *not* complement each other but actually be counterproductive or even harmful.

Also remember that what you do NOT do is important. If you lead a sedentary life, do not expect supplements to greatly improve your health and physical well-being. If you do not give up smoking, you counteract any effects a supplement may provide. The same applies to your choice of food and drink.

One Further Consideration

While such things as diet are discussed in the following chapter, it needs to be mentioned in this chapter within the context of exercise and sport. Diet has always played a role in the training of athletes. Lean body mass and the ability to deliver when necessary are keys to the selection of a diet. Articles such as "Post Long Run Refueling" (Barbich, 2010), "Performance Enhancing with Substance" (Cieciwa, 2010), and "Wine and Dine like a Pro" (Dupré, 2010) are only a few examples of the varied approaches to the combining of athletes, sports, and diet. It is all about the proper amount of carbohydrates, fat, and proteins.

NO can be produced and maintained by the right combination of food within your diet and nutritional intake. If you introduce too much of the wrong fat, it prohibits the production of NO. Research does prove that the wrong type of fat does prevent NO and other helpful enzymes and proteins from doing their job (Luiking, Engelen, and Deutz, 2010). It literally and figuratively will clog your arteries.

When selecting your diet, be sure to consider "cellular nutrition" (Kantor, 2005). This is what the cells of your body will require to continue to operate at their maximum. Healthy and functioning cells have certain needs. This will involve your decision to alter your diet to suit the sport while addressing the demands of your body. Whether you are a bodybuilder or a track-and-field athlete, your endothelial cells will need a diet that includes vitamins A and C. These are antioxidants. They help prevent the breaking down (oxidation) of such free radicals as NO (Marcovitch, 2006). Oxidation prevents or inhibits NO from playing its role in the body. As we know already, a lack of NO is a dangerous condition.

While antioxidants are present in many different fruits and vegetables, they also come in supplement form. Whether you pop them as a pill or eat them is up to you and your trainer and/or medical professional. What you do need to be sure of are the properties. Take care that the antioxidants contain L-arginine, help in NOS, or are at least able to protect the entire process of NO production within the body.

This does not mean you have to omit all foods you enjoy. The next chapter shows that you can still enjoy certain foods you might think were counterproductive to being healthy. For instance, if you add a little wine to your diet, you can actually increase both the production of NO and help improve the functioning of your immune system. One thing is completely clear when considering the production and continuation of NO and its effect on you and the health of your body: nothing except the actual molecular construction of NO is simple.

Conclusion

Exercise does play a crucial role in the ability of the body, particularly the endothelial cells, to manufacture NO. NO is both a by-product of exercising and a factor in promoting improved body health through exercise. NO helps those who exercise regularly to improve their cardiovascular health. It is also a contributing factor in boosting the immune system.

For athletes, a heart and respiratory system that work optimally are essential. An exercise regime helps to improve and maintain enough NO to arrive at this result. While NO is not the only factor, it does contribute substantially to the ability of athletes to perform at their best. This applies to all sports, including bodybuilding. This latter has particularly chosen to embrace the various capabilities of NO.

The bodybuilding sport and industry has chosen to promote NO as a perfect tool for helping you increase lean muscle growth, build up muscle strength and power, and help you work through the pain these actions may involve. NO is served up as a wonder drink, a way to achieve that ripped work naturally.

While NO can and does help in this regard, it does not do so alone. The entire process of obtaining the ideal bodybuilder body is not the sole responsibility of or response to the utilization of NO derived from L-arginine and related arginine substances. Lifestyles must adapt to meet the challenges. In the long run, it is up to you, not NO, to change your current ability to live a long, healthy, and productive life. This holds true whether you are a professional athlete, competitive bodybuilder, or weekend warrior.

6

Saying Yes to No: Diet, Exercise, and Supplements

NITRIC OXIDE IS a fascinating molecule. Researchers are still uncovering what it does and what it can and is possible for it to do. What matters is that NO is proven to be beneficial in so many different aspects. If we ignore its existence, it can result in a lack of NO. In turn, the consequences can be severe health issues.

Rather than dispute what NO does and how exactly it performs, individuals should embrace its existence. They should accept the positive aspects while being aware of the negative. They should also consider how to make sure their body is able to continue to have enough NO on hand.

When someone finally decides to say yes to NO, it is essential to look at ways of ensuring the presence of nitric oxide in the body. There are many ways to accomplish this and improve your overall health while doing so. Yet, in this case, it is best to begin with consideration of that most common characteristic of daily life: diet.

Diet and Nutrition, or You Are What You Eat

It is almost impossible to separate diet from nutrition. Even questionable foods qualify as nutrition of some sort in the most basic sense of the word. When considering improving NO, it is essential to look at those foods containing the amino acid responsible for NO production in the body. This is arginine.

ARGININE AND FOOD

Arginine is both an essential and a non-essential nutrient (Fried, 1999). In other words, it is one your body can produce naturally (non-essential). Arginine is also a nutrient your body is unable to produce, yet still requires for maintaining good health (essential). No matter how you look at it, arginine is the major source of the body's supply of NO. Fortunately, it is found in a wide variety of foods.

If you wish to increase the ability for your body to create NO, consider eating select foods from the following. The first group contains the highest amounts of L-arginine:

- Meat

- Poultry

- Fish and other seafood

- Eggs

- Dairy

- Wild game

These foods contain lower quantities of L-arginine:

- Wheat germ

- Legumes

- Nuts

- Seeds

It is, therefore, rather easy to prepare a meal that tastes good while still being high in arginine. Caldwell Esselstyn offers many delicious suggestions in his book *Prevent and Reverse Heart Disease* (2008). Recipes contain some common foods, including almonds, cashews, salmon, peanuts, wild rice, walnuts, lentils, and peas.

CREATING A MEAL

It is far from difficult for anyone to prepare and actually enjoy a meal designed to boost the levels of NO in your body. Increasing dietary arginine is easy for anyone and everyone. It is not even hard to make finicky food eaters a meal they may actually enjoy. The same is valid for those who are sensitive or allergic, vegetarian, vegan, or even meat-and-potatoes individuals.

From breakfast to lunch to dinner to snacks, arginine-rich foods provide little bother, unless you want to complicate things by making elaborate dishes. Even dessert is available and delicious. Of course, it all depends upon taste and personal preference, but foods containing arginine are nothing if not diverse and accommodating.

For breakfast, satisfy your hunger with oatmeal. This is great for winter. It will also satisfy your body's need for arginine. You could also have eggs or some people's favorite: peanut butter sandwiches.

Many foods high in arginine are acceptable for vegetarian or vegan meals. They can have the oatmeal and may be able to enjoy the peanut butter while ignoring the eggs. They can also cook up an arginine-high meal for either lunch or dinner consisting of soybeans, tofu, lentils, winter squash, and/or garbanzo beans. Others can continue to eat turkey and other meat products, although wild game is the meat containing the greatest amount of arginine.

The meal may be satisfying, but what about afterwards? No one looking to keep their NO production high need ever fear they have to go without dessert. While fruits are low in arginine, chocolate—yes, chocolate—is not (Maroon, 2009). You can enjoy a piece of this delectable treat without guilt— you are doing it for the good of your heart, your respiratory system, your immune system, and even your digestive tract. Just make sure the chocolate is pure and dark.

For a snack, consider the doubly blessed pumpkin seed. Pumpkin seeds are rich in L-arginine and also contain L-citrulline (Roizen, et. al., 2008). Alternatively, you can munch on foods containing almonds, walnuts, macadamia nuts, pistachios, hazelnuts, sunflower seeds, sesame seeds, and even pecans. For those who are hardcore meat eaters, why not enjoy pork rinds?

To end off the meal in a satisfying yet tasty fashion, choose cocoa (only the finest and darkest) or red wine. Both substances are high in arginine. In fact, research into wine indicates that red wine is beneficial in several ways.

As a factor in the formation of NO, it helps in the prevention of hardening of the arteries (Maroon, 2009; Gresele, et. al, 2008). It can also be a preventive measure against cancer.

COMMONALITIES

The foods high in L-arginine have several things in common. Some of them fall into the omega-3 fatty acid group. This classification of food is healthy for you on different levels. The release of L-arginine happens to be one of them. Omega-3 is also reported to stabilize the beating of your heart (Roizen, et. al., 2008).

One further point to consider is significant if you are having a down day. Many of these foods qualify as "happy foods." They relieve stress. They relax the body and elevate the mood. This latter characteristic is particularly true of chocolate (Sears, et. al., 2010). Yet if you truly enjoy wine and imbibe in enough of it, you will also reach that certain stage where life is wonderful.

CAUTION

Whatever your choice, be sure you cook everything in an arginine-friendly oil. Choose only from vegetable oils. Keep them pure. An excellent choice is olive oil. Virgin olive oil is considered one of the best choices to help you obtain arginine. Not only will vegetable oils help in the production of NO within the body, they will also prevent you from putting in your system one of the biggest enemies of NO production: fat.

FOOD AS AN ENEMY OF NO PRODUCTION

If you wish to avoid clogging and hardening of the arteries, you need to stop consuming junk food and other products high in fat, carbohydrates, and unprocessed sugar. While lean meats help in the production of NO, fatty eats have the opposite effect. In fact, fat actually decreases the ability of the endothelial cells to manufacture NO (Esselstyn, 2008). Fat cells even block the release of NO into the blood vessels, resulting ultimately in various cardiovascular problems, including heart and stroke.

If you want to avoid the foods that slow down, inhibit, or even prevent the formation, release, or amount of NO, take a look at this basic list. It contains some of the major enemies of NO.

- Luncheon meats

- Fatty meats and any high-fat diet. Research clearly indicates the problems created by diets high in fats. The result is impaired manufacturing of NO (Luiking, et. al., 2010).

- Baked goods

- Fried fast food

- Palm oil

- Coconut oil

- White processed food

- Foods with "simple sugars" as an ingredient, e.g. those containing corn, malt, rice, or maple syrup. If you read the labels of soft drinks and most sweet, processed food, a prominent ingredient will be HFCS—high fructose corn syrup. While NO helps decrease inflammation, HFCS can actually help increase it (Sears, et. al., 2010).

These foods are helpful only in adding to your waistline and providing a messy layer comprised of carbohydrates and fats called plaque. Fats are also linked to high cholesterol. In part, this is the result of the body's inability to create the correct amount of NO.

Exercise

As discussed in the chapter on NO and sports, it is remarked how NO production increases with exercise. Exercise is a catalyst in the manufacture and release of NO. Regular exercise is described as having specific beneficial effects on many systems, particularly the cardiovascular system (Maiorana, et. al, 2003). Exercise has also been found to contribute to the regulation of the vascular system through the manufacture of NO (Shen, et. al., 1995).

NO also provides the flight-or-fight response that comes in certain types of exercise/training. It works with the adrenal glands to produce the adrenaline you need to work through your exercises. In doing so, exercise acts in a positive fashion, creating NO to arrive at the right moment and in the right amount.

However, as some sports medicine professionals and researchers have noted, exercise on certain levels can exhaust the body's ability to recover quickly (Barbarich, 2010). NO compensates for that. An infusion of NO helps the body's immune system recover more quickly. It also works to reduce inflammation and improve the healing process.

Supplements

'Supplement' is a simple enough word. It refers to anything additional you add to your diet. The intent is to provide the body with something it is lacking—to help address a deficiency. Vitamins and mineral supplements are common in modern-day life. They are part of what we see necessary as a means of coping with stress and replacing what we may be missing from our diet. They fulfill various types of real or perceived shortages within our bodies. Iron supplements, in particular, find their way onto the shelves and in the medicine cabinets of women, pregnant or not.

If you cannot obtain enough arginine in your daily diet, you can turn to supplements. In general, however, arginine supplements are more frequently produced and marketed for those who are interested in building up their body. They are also used in the sporting world as a means of helping the body recover quickly from various health and potential health issues.

FORMAT

Arginine supplements often come in powdered form. Powdered arginine contains both L-arginine and L-ornithine. The latter is also an amino acid. The two, combined with other ingredients, are sold as a power formula (Fried, 1999). The various components make a shake or drink that is intended to aid the body in releasing NO by giving the endothelial cells what they need to manufacture it: L-arginine. These, in turn, are intended to help the body arrive at means through which you obtain a specific goal. In bodybuilding, that means one thing: a sculpted, powerful, lean, mean, bodybuilding machine.

The claims for L-arginine supplements rest on the ability of NO to perform all of its different tasks in the cardiovascular, endocrine, and immune system. As mentioned in the previous chapter, ads refer to the ability of NO supplements to help you build up strength. Various manufacturers and retailers stress the recuperative powers the body will soon possess after regular use. They point out how the use of NO-based power nutritional supplements will increase an individual's endurance.

While, arguably, many of the claims made are legitimate, the results will always vary. The ability of NO to create from every single body the perfect specimen is dubious. Genetic make-up, individual habits, and other factors including age, gender, dedication to the goal, and health will all influence the stated and desirable result.

Other Means of Boosting Your NO

There are other ways to improve your formation and circulation of NO. Among the more popular suggestions are breathing exercises. Deep breathing is perceived as a means through which the release of NO is stimulated. This usually occurs through the nostrils.

To practice this exercise, which has the benefits of helping you stay calm and reduce the level of stress, does not require any special equipment or products. You can practice deep breathing anywhere. Sit or stand, it makes little difference. What does matter is breathing deeply using your nostrils.

This may sound and look funny—drawing interested or disgusted glances from anyone nearby—but it is effective. Deep breathing, according to several experts, helps NO residing in the nostrils and nasal passages to set forth in its role as a dilator of blood vessels in your lungs, improving them in their functional capacity (Roizen, et. al., 2008).

A further suggestion if you feel your NO needs a boost is to read. Reading is good for stimulating NO in the brain. The only catch is it needs to be challenging reading. A romantic novel, mystery, or pulp paperback may not cut it. What you will require is something heavy. You need something as stimulating and challenging to your brain as, say, a book on nitric oxide. Read on and maybe you will not only learn more about NO, but also increase the amount inside your brain. This, in turn, will provide you with more stimulation—perhaps enough to finish reading this book.

Conclusion

The ability of NO to perform so many tasks within the body makes it one of the more essential gases within the system. It is a natural process created within to perform tasks that are in contrast to its size. NO is an active component of the endocrine, immune, and cardiovascular systems. It contributes to the flow of blood, hormones, and disease-fighting bodies. It can act swiftly. It can react with immediate deadly force or organize a campaign of annihilation.

To manage it is a balancing act for the endothelial cells. They need to obtain L-arginine to manufacture the basic tool: NO. With the help of the eNOS, the endothelium can do so. iNOS and other variations also strive to keep their part of the NO production equation going.

Yet without the proper input of the owner of the body, it can come to naught. Food containing arginine must make its way into the system. Consuming meat, fish, roots, and certain nuts and seeds is an excellent start. Throw in a few pieces of high-quality, decadent, pure dark chocolate. Next add a glass of wine. These last are truly food for the gods and, thankfully, for NO.

Exercise always helps. It encourages the release of NO into the various systems. This is particularly true of the cardiovascular and respiratory systems. Exercise is also helpful in stimulating the manufacture of NO in the immune system.

Eliminate such factors as overeating unsuitable foods—those high in sugar and fats. Stop smoking. In fact, do everything that medical professionals and health gurus tell you will result in a healthy and long life. Much of what you then practice will result in the ongoing production of NO. In fact, without thinking about it, you may already be leading the kind of lifestyle that results in the creation of the right amount of NO. If this is so, sit back. You may even ignore the next chapter. Its focus is on what can possibly happen when good NO goes bad.

7

No Gone Bad: The Deleterious Effects of No

NO BOOK ON NO would be complete without at least a consideration of its "bad side." Indeed, many researchers and medical professionals have noted that NO does present some problems. Over the time period since the knowledge of NO has been in existence, it has been a subject of what seem like endless study. For most researchers, it has been assigned protective and beneficial as well as toxic roles (Miranda, et. al., 2010). There is, as Jugdutt (2009) suggested, a "duality" about the molecule.

Yet, in certain incidences, NO has to be toxic. If it is to work with and within the immune system, for example, NO must be deadly. It needs to kill off, annihilate, and completely destroy any invaders. If it fails to do so, the cancer or infection will spread. Damage will occur. The body will become ill and the invaders may well spread their own toxins to other parts of the anatomy. Yet a single question continues to form the basis of certain types of NO research: How much NO is toxic to the human host?

QUESTIONS CONCERNING NO

Since the discovery of NO within the human body, it has been the focus of controversy. While much stemmed from the obvious deleterious effects of

NO in its role as smog, others focused on other aspects and concerns. The complexity of the role played by NO in biological processes has resulted in an ongoing controversy about it (Lee, et. al., 2010). Some areas have, naturally, received more than a little attention in determining what NO can and cannot accomplish as either beneficial or detrimental.

These are related to other specific concerns about using NO: the dosage and levels. Researchers have become increasingly interested in answering questions concerning this characteristic. Common questions researchers ask themselves include:

- How much NO should be in the body?

- How low are the levels when NO fails to perform its task?

- How high are the levels when NO "goes rogue"?

- How much NO is too little?

- How much NO is too much?

The following sections will attempt to shed a tiny bit of light on the little that researchers have discovered. It will consider what they have found and what it actually says about NO. First, however, you need to understand how the levels of NO may become elevated.

CAUSES OF HIGH LEVELS OF NO

There are several ways the levels of NO can become higher than the norm. During laboratory research, the levels of NO are artificially enhanced using drugs. The levels can also be increased through the use of inhalers or respiratory devices. Individuals tend to perhaps dangerous higher levels of NO through other means.

We have previously noted how you can increase the amount of NO in your body by eating foods high in NO. The addition of supplements to your diet can also result in increased NO levels. Yet there are also ways NO can become dangerously high in your system. These range from taking prescription and non-prescription drugs to the body's own immune response.

Among various factors in raising the presence of NO in your body are:

- Using antihistamines

- A chronic lack of oxygen—this will trigger the release of NO to compensate for the problem.

- Iron deficiency

- Carbon monoxide. Breathing this substance in may be unhealthy for you in more than one way.

It is important to understand the factors behind the production of NO in high amounts. This will result in the ability of the medical profession to reduce and control the levels in order to prevent or address various existing and potential health issues.

Dosage and Levels

A major question for researchers is "How much?" This can refer to related but separate aspects of the amount of something within the system. Dosage indicates the amount of a substance an individual takes. Level refers to the amount of a substance within the system. For example, if all factors are optimum, when you increase the dosage, you also increase the levels of the substance within the body.

WHY INCREASE THE DOSAGE AND RAISE THE LEVELS?

Raising the levels of NO is part of a strategy by some individuals to improve the ability of their body to perform a variety of functions. After a race, a competitor may want to ingest more arginine to speed up the process of healing. Adding NO to the body will boost the immune system, which, in turn, will help the individual heal.

Bodybuilders will also try to raise the levels of NO within their bodies. They will take NO in supplement form. The purpose of this is to help increase the ability of their body to look, perform, and heal better. If they are using NO as fast as they are putting it into their body, there is little chance of the levels reaching a questionable level—a level where serious damage could and has occurred. To put it mildly, because of the extent of the endothelium and the extensive applications required of NO, any malfunctioning, any levels that fall below the normal requirements of the body mechanism, can be disastrous for all involved (von Hachling, 2004; Bryan, et. al., 2011).

Can Dosage and Levels Be Too Low or Too High?

Researchers have been experimenting with the effect of low and high dosages and levels for decades. They are quite aware of what happens when the levels of NO fall below what is necessary for optimum body function. The lack of NO function has been connected with various deleterious effects. Previous chapters have noted that when NO is not present to perform its tasks, the body becomes affected by various malfunctions and diseases.

The immune system may "go down," leaving the individual vulnerable to immune-deficiency diseases, cancers, and other infections, both serious and minor. A person may suffer from various cardiovascular system problems, such as high blood pressure, hardening of the arteries, a stroke, heart attack, or chronic heart failure (Von Hachling, et. al., 2004).

Studies also look at what occurs when the levels rise too high. This is when the issue becomes less straightforward and researchers begin to divide themselves into various camps. It does not help that in many instances, NO is not acting alone. The many different variables involved in the process of healing or accomplishing a function are rarely as simple. The body is a complex organism and, while NO is a simple molecule, it does not work alone in performing its various functions. In other words, it is not just a question of "just add NO and stir."

THE VERDICT OF THE EXPERTS

To date, the results have been varied. Some researchers argue that there cannot be too much NO. Others disagree. The majority, however, seem to follow the premise that a little NO is a beautiful thing. Too much NO can be harmful (Napoli, et. al., 2010).

Studies by various researchers seem to back up these findings. Work by Jugdutt (2004) indicates that small, continuous doses are highly beneficial to alleviate or prevent issues concerning the regular and necessary flow of blood. This helps out various problems, including those affecting the cardiovascular and immune systems. However, his research indicates that high doses can result in hypertension.

Napoli (2010) agrees. In his studies, he formed the opinion that small amounts of NO are beneficial. They contribute to normal physiological process of the body or homeostasis. The right amount of NO ensures the blood flows and does not stick. When too much is released, the result is possible cell damage or even death (apoptosis).

Other research involving the role of NO in decreasing swollen joints found similar results. If NO was present and activated in small concentrations, it helped decrease the inflammation and swelling. If concentrations of NO were high, however, the gas molecule actually appeared to hinder the healing process (Butler, et. al, 2003). In some cases, NO could actually increase the problem, exasperating inflammation, helping with the spread of cancerous tissue and tumors, as well as other immune system disorders and diseases.

Studies of the relationship between certain eye problems and high amounts of NO also indicated a negative result. High levels of NO actually seemed to produce chronic open angle glaucoma or COAG. They also have appeared to be related to cases of male infertility, specifically sperm count (European Society for Human Reproduction and Embryology, 2006). Other studies conducted implicate overproduction of NO in the problem of neurodegeneration in the central nervous system (Luiking, Engelsen, and Deutz, 2010).

There is, therefore, one specific fact that substantial numbers of both researchers and medical professionals have agreed upon: too little NO results in serious health issues. Studies and further research by Jugdutt (2004), Bonavida (2010), and Butler (2003) all point to this seemingly inevitable answer to the question about dosage and levels. Yet there are always dissenters to the general theory. This is the result, once again, of the complexity of the processes that make the body function.

Opposing Views

By this time, you should not be surprised that there is an opposing view. Why should NO conform to certain expectations? It is the good/bad dichotomy all over again. In fact, there are at least two views. Essentially, what the researchers are saying is this:

- Too much NO does not cause or help in the development of diseases.

- While the levels of NO may be high in the system, they are not at fault.

- Increasing the dosage will not increase the problem or health issue, although decreasing the level of NO beneath the required amount will.

- In fact, in some studies, the presence of high amounts of NO in the system was actually described as beneficial.

THE RESEARCH

The research is still ongoing. Among the studies performed on the negative and positive effects too-high levels of NO will have is one conducted by Martin Feelisch (2008). While no study on NO has ever been entirely conclusive—partly being the nature of scientific research and partly because of the nature of NO—this one indicated that too much NO was not the culprit in various illnesses, diseases, and deaths.

In his work on the role of NO in osteoarthritis, Feelisch (2008) examined what the impact of elevated levels of NO would have on the disease. Would too much NO actually contribute to the problem? Were too-high levels of NO actually responsible for triggering osteoarthritis?

The answer was no. Higher levels than normal of NO were not perceived as a direct or indirect cause of the incidence of the disease. Feelisch (2008) based his argument on other factors involved in the process. The argument specifically focuses on the complexity of the processes involving NO. While NO does play a significant role, it is not the only player. There are many other substances that could be at fault.

The argument is quite logical. The body is a complex organism. Furthermore, NO has been proven to be just as complex. It is a mediator, a neurotransmitter, a vasodilator, and a destroyer. It can be both toxic and benign.

The other body of work that supports the concept of high levels of NO being beneficial includes research by the American Thoracic Society (2007). Their studies found that elevated levels of NO within the urine indicated positive results for the individuals in the study. In fact, those with higher levels of NO had a higher level of survival for two related respiratory system problems. NO was a positive indicator of survival for those who had acute respiratory distress syndrome (ARDS) or its precursor, acute lung injury (ALI) [American Thoracic Society, 2007].

It will require further research into all the different aspects of NO before anyone can reach a conclusion on the role higher levels of NO plays in creating, encouraging, or mediating the onset, development, and/or spread of various disorders and diseases.

Conclusion

The levels of NO are dependent upon a variety of factors, including how much arginine you put into the body. The state of health of the endothelium cells is also significant. If this important organism malfunctions, resulting in too little, too much, or even no NO at all, the body will suffer.

Yet the question of how much NO is required to maintain a balance is still debatable. Furthermore, opinions vary as to the issue of whether high levels of NO are harmful or not. While generally it seems that good levels of NO are low levels of NO, this is not always the case.

Research also seems to indicate that the presence of high levels of NO may actually not be toxic to the body. They may be fatal to the invasive element. They may also be indicative that the individual will survive. Perhaps it is the disparity of the measuring tools used. This is one possible answer put forth by Luiking and colleagues (2010). Yet the sometimes contradictory findings seem to be part of the nature of the functions of NO within the body. It is truly dual in all aspects.

8

Conclusion

NO IS AN extremely versatile and significant factor acting in a wide variety of functions within and throughout the human body. While it is a very simple molecule in its biological and chemical structure, it is an integral part of a multitude and variety of biological and medical processes. These range from controlling the flow of the blood stream through the endothelium to acting as a major neurotransmitter. On the one hand, it helps overcome things as diverse as disease-causing cells and infections of the immune system; on the other hand, it is applied to increase sexual potency through overcoming erectile dysfunction.

Consider the magnitude of NO's involvement and possible influence in the diverse processes of human biology. NO has been reported to contribute to the following processes:

- Blood circulation: NO acts within the circulatory system to improve blood circulation. It affects the condition of smooth muscles, causing them to relax. It makes the linings of the vessels slippery and, therefore, prevents the concentration and build-up of such things as plaque. As a result, it decreases or even prevents the risk of such cardiovascular problems as high blood pressure, hardened arteries, stroke, and heart attack.

- Nerve communication: NO acts as a neurotransmitter and messenger. It sends commands off to perform specific functions that help the body perform at its best or to fight off health problems.

- Learning: Although the exact mechanisms are as yet unknown, NO contributes to our ability to learn.

- Memory: NO is also responsible for the brain's ability to remember things. This is more applicable to long-term rather than short-term memory.

- Digestion: As part of the digestive tract, NO works within the stomach lining to help protect it against ulcers.

- Fighting disease: NO plays a definite role within the body's immune system. It works within macrophages, for example, to seek out and destroy disease-causing bacteria and viruses. As a result, it prevents and even eliminates many harmful and potentially life-threatening diseases. It helps decrease inflammation and battles to protect you from any health problems.

- Sexual problems: NO is renowned for its ability to improve or actually induce sexual performance. It has been clinically proven to help in cases of erectile dysfunction. This forever will carve its niche in the annals of male history.

This is quite an extensive and impressive list for a Johnny-come-lately discovery.

Research clearly indicates the significance of this highly reactive little molecule. It has discussed it at length in terms of the various interactions involved in production and the roles played by NOS, L-arginine, and citrulline. Diet, exercise, supplements, and other possible sources of NO production have been examined.

Attention has been paid to other areas of research and concern. Since NO is a relatively unknown molecule, this results in extensive research into diverse areas. One area of study focuses on the amounts, levels, and dosages of NO. It looks at whether high or low levels are detrimental.

While no NO is definitely harmful to the body and results in the onset of a variety of disease, the research around the results of too much NO are less clear-cut. Scientists are still searching for an absolute answer to several questions. Prominent among these is the issue of if too much NO is toxic in the body.

The jury is still out. Research has not provided an answer that is capable of addressing all the uses of NO. Since NO is a gas that does not linger, this also complicates matters. Evidence seems to suggest that NO may be both beneficial and toxic in high amounts. This may be the result of the complicated processes involved. It may also be the result of different applications and roles of NO in the system. The methods of measuring NO may also be at fault.

And it is not merely medical application that has chosen to explore the uses of NO. NO has made it into the mainstream. Knowledge of how NO can help improve performance and training has become noticed by various professional and minor sports practitioners and trainers. It has been applied as a means to increase the level of energy and to boost the immune system following strenuous competitions or training sessions.

Where NO has gained a more sensational type of attention is in bodybuilding. It has become integrated in various drinks. Powered forms of L-arginine and other arginine derivatives are consumed by bodybuilders and other enthusiasts of the sport on a daily basis. While little attention is drawn by the mainstream media to the medical applications and implications of using NO, pages upon pages of advertisements and articles extol the use in sport and bodybuilding.

One other popular use for NO has also been widely hailed. This is as a means of addressing the issue of sexual dysfunction among males. While the effect of NO on sperm account is largely ignored in television, in print, or in electronic ads, NO does get a nod—although it is a discreet one—for its role in helping reverse erectile dysfunction.

Truly, NO is multi-faceted. It is the little molecule that could and still can. It is a mighty molecule that may still surprise the world with what it can do.

Glossary

ADMA: The full name is asymmetric dimethylarginine. This refers to a modified amino acid capable of preventing the production of nitric oxide.

ARDS: This is short for acute respiratory distress syndrome. It is a condition of the lungs with a high mortality rate triggered by unknown sources resulting in loss of oxygen in the blood (hypoxaemia).

Adrenal glands: Located just above the kidney, these two glands are responsible for the production of adrenaline and noradrenaline. These two hormones aid with the constriction of the blood vessels in two distinct areas: the skin and the abdomen (barring the intestines).

Antatherogenic: This is a term referring to something that prevents clogging of the arteries.

Angina: This condition characterized by a tightness of the chest, heaviness, or external pressure on the chest is the result of the narrowing of the arteries to the heart, which causes atherosclerosis.

Apoptosis: This refers to the death of a cell in a slow, very controlled, and orchestrated manner. It is death through planning.

Arginine: This is an amino acid found commonly in certain foods that reacts in the endothelial cells to produce nitric oxide and L-citrulline.

Cardiovascular system: This is a system consisting of such life-giving organs as the heart, lungs, arteries, and blood.

Central nervous system: This consists of the brain and the spinal cord. It is one of the most important systems within the body.

Cyclic GMP: A secondary messenger used by nitric oxide to bring about various actions. For example, it creates relaxation within the smooth muscle cells.

Cyclic guanosine monophosphate or cGMP: This is a cyclic nucleotide that acts as both a second messenger and a relaxer of smooth muscles. cGMP in its role as a very powerful vasodilator will cause the blood to flow to the penis, creating an erection.

Cytokine: This small protein is characterized by its ability to interact within the cell, producing, in response to infection, inflammation.

Deposition: The term refers to the formation of a new bone.

Endocrine glands: These form part of the overall endocrine system, although the two terms are often interchangeable. The endocrine glands are responsible for producing hormones that direct the body to start, speed up, slow down, and even cease certain actions. Among the glands related to NO activities are the adrenal glands, the pancreas, and the hypothalamus.

Endocrine system: This important system within the body consists of several important and diverse glands. It is a control center or system for the entire body. The glands are found in separate areas of the body. Among the more important glands involved in the processes of NO are the hypothalamus, the adrenals, and the pancreas. Important organs include the liver, the gonads, the kidneys, and the heart.

Endothelial cells: These are the cells that make up the endothelium.

Endothelium: This is a single carpet lining of flat cells that line the inner section of a blood vessel.

Endothelium-derived relaxing factor (EDRF): This is identical to the molecule known as nitric oxide or NO. It acts as a messenger to the vascular muscle to relax.

Essential nutrients: This refers to carbohydrates, fats, minerals, proteins, vitamins, and water, which are essential for normal function, growth, and maintenance of the body. The only source is food, as the body is unable to make them or cannot produce them in sufficient quantities necessary to retain a healthy norm.

Gastrointestinal tract: This refers to what is often called the digestive system. It consists of the mouth, throat, gullet, stomach, small and big intestines, and the rectum. Its purpose is to handle digestion. This includes both taking in nutrition and removing waste from the body.

Gonads: These are sex glands. They produce either testes or ovaries.

HGH: This is short for human growth hormone. This hormone, released by the pituitary gland, is responsible for the growth of cells within the body. A banned substance for use in most sports, it is considered by some a clue to achieving a longer life.

Hypothalamus: This is located in the forebrain. Its main purpose is to perform as a thermo-regulator or body-temperature controller.

Immune system: This is not a centralized system within the body. It consists of various agents acting throughout the body in response to and to prevent infection and various diseases, disorders, and related health problems.

Isoform: This is a term referring to different forms of the same protein. In NOS, for example, it is NOS1, NOS2, and NOS3.

L-arginine: The term is used interchangeably with arginine by many authors.

Lipophilic: This means that the substance is attracted to fats.

Macrophage: This refers to the small cells that are scavengers. As an integral part of the immune system, macrophages seek out and destroy invading harmful microbes/germs.

Mitogen: An agent in the process called mitosis.

Mitosis: This refers to the splitting and multiplying of cells.

Necrosis: This refers to the death of a cell in a limited fashion.

Nitric oxide: Referred to as NO or EDRF, this is a molecule formed by the uniting of one nitrogen and one oxygen molecule. It is now known to play a crucial role in many areas of the human body, including the endocrine, immune, and cardiovascular systems.

Non-essential nutrient: This refers to a substance such as a protein, fat, or mineral that the body is able to create or produce within itself.

NOS: This is nitric oxide synthase. This refers to the enzyme responsible for producing NO within the blood cell.

Pancreas: The pancreas is found just below the stomach. The pancreatic duct attaches this organ to the small intestine. Two hormones originate in this gland: insulin and glucagon. Both act to control blood sugar levels.

Plaque: When platelets and fat molecules gather and become stuck together in place, this is called plaque. Essentially, it is a build-up of platelets that occurs when the blood vessels are narrow or not slick enough to prevent clumping.

Platelet: These are small particles located within the blood that, when joined together, form blood clots.

Pulmonary: Related to the lungs.

Resorption: This is the term for bone depletion. If followed by the process of bone deposition, it is a healthy and natural process.

Respiratory system: The respiratory system consists of the airways, lungs and the respiratory muscles. Oxygen and carbon dioxide are exchanged by diffusion between blood and the external environment.

Smooth muscle: This refers to the appearance of the muscles as smooth. They are found throughout the body of most mammals, comprising the walls of the blood vessels.

Tumor: The term actually refers to any form of swelling. It is usually restricted to any type of swelling resulting from the uncontrolled growth of the cells.

Vasodilator: A substance that is capable of causing the blood vessels to dilate.

Vascular smooth muscle: This is the muscle that forms the walls of the blood vessels. If it contracts, blood flow is restricted. If it relaxes, blood flow increases.

Vasculature: This is comprised of the blood vessels that conduct the blood within the body.

References

American Thoracic Society (February 20, 2007). "Higher Nitric Oxide Levels Increase Survival For Acute Lung Injury And Acute Respiratory Distress Syndrome Patients." *ScienceDaily*. Retrieved August 1, 2011, from http://www.sciencedaily.com /releases/2007/02/070201082600.htm

Aaronson, P. I., and Ward, J. P. T., 2010. *The Cardiovascular System at a Glance*. Massachusetts: Blackwell Pub.

Ahker, D., and Bassengo, E., 2004. "Statins and the Role of Nitric Oxide in Chronic Heart Failure." In Jugdutt (ed)

Barbich, Bobbi, 2010."Post-Long Run Refueling." *Canadian Running*, Sept./Oct.

Bonavida, Benjamin (ed), 2010. *Nitric Oxide and Cancer. Prevention and Therapy*. New York: Springer

Bonavida, Benjamin, 2010. "Novel Therapeutic Applications of Nitric Oxide in the Inhibition of Tumor Malignancy and Reversal of Resistance." In L. Ignarro (ed)

Bonavida, B., Faritakis, S., Huerta-Yepezi, S., Vega, M. I., Jazirehi, A. R., and Berenson, J., 2010. "Nitric Oxide Donors are a New Class of Anti-cancer Therapies for the Reversal of Resistance and Inhibition of Metastasis." In Bonavida (ed)

Bryan, Nathan S. (ed), 2010. *Food, Nutrition and the Nitric Oxide Pathway: Biochemistry and Bioactivity*. Destech Pub.: Pennsylvania

Bryan, N.S, and Loscalzo, J., 2011. "Introduction." In *Nitrite and Nitrate in Human Health and Disease*. Bryan and Loscalzo (eds), New York

Bryan, N.S., and Loscalzo, J., 2011. *Nitrite and Nitrate in Human Health and Disease*. New York: Humana Press

Bryan, N.S., and Murad, Ferid, 2010. "What is Nitric Oxide?" in Bryan & Loscalzo (ed)

Burgaud, J. L., Ongini, E., and Del Soldato, P., 2002. "Nitric Oxide Releasing Drugs: A Novel Class of Effective and Safe Therapeutic Agents." *Annals of the New York Academy of Science*. May (962): 360-71

Butler, Anthony, and Nicholson, Rosslyn, 2003. *Life, Death and Nitric Oxide*. Cambridge: RSC

Cheng, R., Ridnow, L. A., Glynn, S. A., Switzer, C. H., Flores-Santana, W., Hussain, P., Thomas, D. D., Ambs, S., Harris, C., and Wink, D. A., 2010. "Nitric Oxide and Cancer: An Overview." In Bonavida (ed)

Cieciwa, Jordan. 2010. "Performance Enhancing with Substance." *Canada Fitness*: October/November.

Clark, Shannon, 2010. "6 Vein-popping Reasons to use Nitric Oxide Supplements." Retrieved From http://www.bodybuilding.com/fun/6-reasons-use-nitric-oxide.htm

Cooke, John, and Zimmer, J., 2003. *The Cardiovascular Cure*. New York: Broadway Books

Desai, K. M., Sessa, W. C., and Vane, J. R., 1991. "Involvement of Nitric Oxide in the Reflex Relaxation of the Stomach to Accommodate Food or Fluid." *Nature*. 351: 477-479

Dunlap, T., Abdul-Hay, S. O., Chandasema, R. E. P., Hagos, G. K., Sinha, V., Wang, H., and Thatcher, G. R. J., 2008. "Nitrates and NO-NSAIDS in Cancer Chemoprevention and Therapy: In vitro Evidence Querying the NO Donor or Functionality." *Nitric Oxide* 19(2): 115-124

Dupré, Elyse, 2010. "Wine and Dine like a Pro." *Men's Fitness*: October

Esselstyn, Caldwell B., 2008. *Prevent and Reverse Heart Disease*. New York: Avery

European Society for Human Reproduction and Embryology, 2006. "Sperm DNA damaged by high levels of nitric oxide." Retrieved From http://www.rxpgnews.com/urology/Sperm_DNA_damaged_by_high_levels_of_nitric_oxide_4514_4514.shtml

Feelisch, Martin, 2008. "The Chemical Biology of Nitric Oxide—An Outsider's Reflections about its Role in Osteoarthritis." *Osteoarthritis and Cartilage*. Volume 16, supp. 2: S3-313

Fried, Robert, and Merrell, Woodson C., 1999. *The Arginine Solution*. New York: Warner Books

Fukato, Jon M., Cho, J. Y., and Switzer, C. H., 2000. "The Chemical Properties of Nitric Oxide and Related Nitrogen Oxides." In Ignarro (ed)

Ganong, William F., 2005. *Review of Medical Physiology*. New York: Lange Medical Books.

Garbán, H. J., 2010. "Breaking Resistance: The Role of Nitric Oxide in the Sensitization of Cancer Cells to Chemo and Immune Therapy." In Bonavida (ed)

Gresele, Paolo, Pignatelli, P., Guglielmini, G., Carnevale, R., Mezzasoma, A. M., Ghiselli, A., Momi, S., and Violi, F., 2008. "Resveratol, at Concentrations Attainable with Moderate Wine Consumption Stimulates Human Platelet Nitric Oxide Production." *J. Nutrition*, Sept: 1602-1608

Guo, X., Oldham, M. J., Kleinman, M. T., Phalen, R. F., and Hassab, G. S., 2006. "Effect of Cigarette Smoking on Nitric Oxide, Structural, and Mechanical Properties of Mouse Arteries." *American Journal of Physiology: Heart and Circulatory Physiology* 291 (5): H2354-H2361

Hartmut G., Knauer, N., Büscher, R., Hübner, R., Drazen, J. M., and Ratjen, F., 2000. "Airway Nitric Oxide Levels in Cystic Fibrosis Patients are Related to a Polymorphism in the Neuronal Nitric Oxide Synthase Gene." *American Journal of Respiratory Critical Care Medicine*, 162, (6): 2172-2176

Hirst, D. G., aAnd Robson, T., 2010. "Nitric Oxide: Monotherapy or Sensitizer to Conventional Cancer Treatments." In Bonavida (ed)

Hukkanen, Mika V.J., and Dolak, Julia (ed), 1998. *Nitric Oxide in Bone and Joint Disease*. Cambridge: Cambridge University Press

Ignarro, Louis (ed), 2000. *Biology and Pathology*. San Diego, California: Elsevier Press

Ignarro, Louis, 2000. "Introduction and Overview." In Ignarro (ed)

Ignarro, Louis J. (ed), 2010. *Nitric Oxide: Biology and Pathology Second Edition*. San Diego, California: Elsevier Press

Ignarro, Louis J., 2008. *No More Heart Disease. How Nitric Oxide Can Prevent— Even Reverse—Heart Disease and Stroke*. New York: St. Martin's Press

Jugdutt, B. I. (ed), 2004. *The Role of Nitric Oxide in Heart Failure*. Boston: Kluwer Academic Pub.

Jugdutt, B. I., 2004. "Nitric Oxide in Heart Failure: Friend or Foe." In Jugdutt (ed)

Kantor, Marissa, 2005. "Nitric Oxide. The New Hero of Human Biology." *Psychology Today*, February 8

MacNaughton, W. K., Cirino, G., and Wallace, J. L., 1989. "Stomach Endotheliun-derived Relaxing Factor (Nitric Oxide) has Protective Action in the Stomach." *Life Sciences* 45 (20):1869-1876

Maroon, Joseph, 2009. *The Longevity Factor: How Resvertol and Red Wine Activate Genes for a Longer and Healthier Life*. New York: Atria Books

Lee, Y. C., Kim, S.-R., Jo, E.-K., Pae, H.-O., and Chung, H.T., 2010. "Nitric Oxide in Airway Inflammation." In Ignarro (ed)

Luiking, Y. C., Engelen, Mariëlle P.K.J., and Deutz, N.E.P., 2010. "Regulation of Nitric Oxide Production in Health and Disease." *Current Opinion Clinical Nutrition Metabolic Care*, 13(1): 97–104

Maiorana, A., O'Driscoll, G., Taylor, R., and Green, D., 2003. "Exercise and the Nitric Oxide Vasodilator System." *Sports Medicine* 33(14): 1013-1035

Marcovitch, Harvey, 2006. *Black's Medical Dictionary 41st edition*. Lanham, Maryland: Scarecrow Press

Miranda, K. M., Espey, M. G., Jourd'heuil, D., Grisham, M. B., Fukuto, J. M., Feelisch, M., and Wink, D. A., 2000. "The Chemical Biology of Nitric Oxide." In Ignarro (ed)

Moncada, Salvador, and Higgs, Annie, 1993. "L-Arginine-Nitric Oxide Pathway." *New England Journal of Medicine* 329 (Dec.): 2002-2012

Napoli, Claude, Crimini, E., Williams-Ignarro, S., de Nigris, Filimeno, and Ignarro, L.J., 2010. "Nitric Oxide in Vascular Damage and Regeneration." In Ignarro (ed)

Readers' Digest, 2011. *Disease Free*. Montreal: Readers' Digest Association

Roizen, M. F., and Oz, M.C., 2008. *You, the Owner's Manual*. New York: Collins

Rushton, Lynette (ed), 2004. *The Endocrine System*. Philadelphia: Chelsea House

ScienceDaily. Retrieved July 29, 2011, from http://www.sciencedaily.com / releases/2008/11/081126133403.htm

Sears, Wm., and Sears, M., 2010. *Prime-Time Health*. New York: Little and Brown

Shen, W., Zhang, X., Shao, G. Wolin, M. S., Sessa, W., and Hintze, H., 1995. "Nitric Oxide Production and NO Synthase Gene Expression Contribute to Vascular Regulation during Exercise." *Medical Science of Sports Exercise*. 27 (Aug.): 8: 1125-1134

Su, Y., Han, W., Giraldo, C., De Lio, Y., and Block, E. R., 1998. "Effect of Cigarette Smoke Extract on nitric Oxide Synthase in Pulmonary Artery Endothelial Cells." *American Journal of Respiratory Cell and Molecular Biology.* 19 (5): 819-825

Thomas, D. D., Flores-Santana, W., Switzer, C. H., Wink, D. A., and Ridnour, L. A., 2010. "Determinants of Nitric Oxide Chemistry: Impact of Cell Signaling Processes." In Ignarro (ed)

Tierney, L. M., McPhee, S. J., and Papadakis, M. A., 2006. *Current Medical Diagnosis and Treatment, 45th Edition.* New York: Lange Medical Books

Vallance, Patrick, and Moncada, Salvador, 1998. "A Brief Overview of the Biology of Nitric Oxide." In Hukkanen and Dolak (eds)

Von Hachling, S., Anker, S., and Bassenger, E., 2004. "Statins and the Role of Nitric Oxide in Chronic Heart Failure." In Jugdutt (ed)